OVERCOMING ANXIETY DISORDERS

A PRACTICAL GUIDE TO MANAGING STRESS AND WORRY

LUCAS HOFFMAN

COPYRIGHT

DEDICATION

To my family and friends, who have supported and encouraged me throughout this journey. Your love and support have been very important to me and have helped me keep going through the hard times. Thank you for believing in me and for being my rock. This book is dedicated to you.

TABLE OF CONTENTS

INTRODUCTION

Anxiety is a normal human emotion that everyone experiences at some point in their lives. However, when anxiety becomes excessive and persistent, it can interfere with daily activities and have a negative impact on overall well-being. That's where *"Overcoming Anxiety Disorders: A Practical Guide to Managing Stress and Worry"* comes in. This book is meant to give people practical, evidence-based ways to deal with and get rid of anxiety.

Anxiety can look like panic attacks, phobias, social anxiety, and generalized anxiety disorder, among other things. The guide will cover the different types of anxiety and their symptoms, so readers can better understand what they are experiencing.

One of the most important parts of this guide is that it focuses on mindfulness and ways to relax. Meditation and yoga, which are both mindful practices, have been shown to help people feel less anxious and stressed. The guide will tell people step-by-step how to use mindfulness and relaxation techniques to deal with anxiety.

Cognitive Behavioral Therapy (CBT) is another evidence-based approach that has been shown to be effective in reducing anxiety. The guide will explain how CBT works and provide readers with tools to identify and challenge negative thoughts and beliefs that contribute to anxiety.

Exercise and nutrition play a crucial role in mental health. The guide will discuss the link between physical activity and mental health and provide tips on how to incorporate exercise and healthy eating habits into daily life to manage anxiety.

Medications and therapy are other options for treating anxiety. The guide will explain the different types of medications used to treat anxiety and provide guidance on how to find a therapist and the benefits of therapy.

The guide will also talk about how to deal with panic disorder, phobias, social anxiety disorder, and generalized anxiety disorder.

Building resilience and developing a support network are important components of managing anxiety. The guide will help people build resilience and support networks that will help them deal with stress and hard times.

The guide will also discuss setting goals, creating a plan to manage anxiety, and providing tips on how to identify and avoid relapse triggers.

Finally, the guide will provide additional resources and support options for those who are struggling with anxiety.

Overall, this guide is meant to be a useful tool for anyone who wants to deal with and lessen anxiety. It gives readers a variety of tools and strategies to help them understand and get rid of their anxiety so they can live a happier, more fulfilling life.

WHAT IS ANXIETY DISORDER

Anxiety disorder is a broad term for a group of mental health conditions that involve excessive, persistent, and irrational worry or fear about everyday things. Anxiety can manifest in many different ways and be experienced as a range of symptoms, such as physical, emotional, and behavioral ones. Anxiety disorders are among the most common mental health disorders, affecting millions of people worldwide.

Common symptoms of anxiety disorders include the following:

- Feelings of unease, restless, or tense.
- Feelings of impending danger, panic, or dread.
- Having a faster heart rate.
- Rapid breathing (hyperventilation).
- Sweating.
- Trembling.
- Feeling exhausted or feeble.
- Having difficulty concentrating or thinking about anything other than the current stress.
- Having difficulty sleeping.
- Having gastrointestinal (GI) issues.
- Having difficulties managing worry.
- Having a strong desire to avoid situations that cause worry.

Anxiety disorders can manifest in different forms and types, such as:

1. Generalized Anxiety Disorder (GAD): GAD is characterized by excessive and unrealistic worry or fear about everyday situations. People with GAD may worry about a wide range of topics such as their health, work, relationships, or financial situation. They may also experience physical symptoms such as muscle tension, fatigue, and restlessness.

2. Panic Disorder: People with panic disorder have panic attacks, which are sudden, intense feelings of fear or discomfort that happen often. People often have physical symptoms like a fast heartbeat, sweating, shaking, and trouble breathing when they have a panic attack.

3. Social Anxiety Disorder: Social Anxiety disorder is characterized by excessive self-consciousness and fear of social situations. People with social anxiety disorder may feel extremely self-conscious in social situations and worry about being judged or rejected by others. They may also experience physical symptoms such as blushing, sweating, or shaking in social situations.

4 Phobias: Phobias are excessive and irrational fears of specific objects or situations. People with phobias may experience intense fear or panic when they encounter the object or situation they fear, and may go to great lengths to avoid it.

5. Obsessive-Compulsive Disorder (OCD): OCD is characterized by persistent unwanted thoughts, known as obsessions, and repetitive behaviors or mental acts, known as compulsions. People with OCD may feel compelled to perform certain actions repeatedly in order to alleviate the anxiety caused by their obsessions.

6. Post-Traumatic Stress Disorder (PTSD): PTSD is a mental health disorder that can develop after a person experiences or witnesses a traumatic event. People with PTSD may experience flashbacks, nightmares, and avoidance of reminders of the traumatic event.

7. Separation Anxiety Disorder (SAD): SAD is a type of anxiety disorder that causes people to worry too much and for too long about being away from home or a loved one. It is typically diagnosed in children and adolescents, but can also occur in adults. SAD can cause significant distress and impairment in social, academic, and occupational functioning.

8. Selective Mutism: Selective Mutism is characterized by an inability to speak in certain social situations, despite the ability to speak in other situations. It is usually diagnosed in children and young people who are otherwise able to communicate in other settings.

9. Body Dysmorphic Disorder (BDD): This is a condition in which a person worries too much about flaws they see in their own bodies. People with BDD may engage in repetitive behaviors such as mirror checking, skin picking, or excessive grooming.

10. Illness Anxiety Disorder (Hypochondria): Illness Anxiety Disorder is characterized by excessive fear of having a serious illness despite medical reassurance. People with Illness Anxiety Disorder may have a preoccupation with their health and may be excessively worried about having a serious illness, even when there is no medical evidence to support it.

Anxiety disorders can be treated, and a mix of therapy, medication, and self-help techniques can help people deal with their anxiety. If you think you might have an anxiety disorder, it's important to get professional help and work with a qualified therapist to come up with a treatment plan that fits your needs.

Now, we would go into much detail about each of the above sets of anxiety disorders, looking at the symptoms, potential causes, and their risk factors.

1. Generalized Anxiety Disorder (GAD)

Generalized Anxiety Disorder (GAD) is a type of anxiety disorder characterized by excessive and unrealistic worry or fear about everyday situations. People with GAD may worry about a wide range of topics, such as their health, work, relationships, or financial situation. They may also experience physical symptoms such as muscle tension, fatigue, and restlessness. GAD is a chronic condition that can last for months or even years if left untreated.

Symptoms

Symptoms of GAD typically include

- Persistent worrying or anxiety about a variety of everyday events or activities.
- Difficulty controlling or reducing worry
- Restlessness, feeling keyed up or on edge
- Fatigue
- Difficulty concentrating or mind going blank
- Irritability
- Muscle tension
- Sleep disturbance

GAD can interfere with daily activities and make it difficult for people to function at home, work, or school. People with GAD may also have trouble sleeping and may have other physical symptoms like headaches, stomach problems, or muscle aches.

Causes

The exact cause of GAD is not known, but it is thought to be related to a combination of genetic, environmental, and psychological factors. GAD is often linked to other mental health problems, like depression, panic disorder, and drug abuse.

Risk Factors

Generalized Anxiety Disorder (GAD) is a complex condition that can be influenced by a combination of genetic, environmental, and psychological factors. Some of the risk factors associated with GAD include:

- **Genetics:** There is some evidence to suggest that GAD may run in families, and that certain genetic variations may increase the risk of developing the disorder.
- **Trauma or stress**: Trauma, such as experiencing a natural disaster, combat, or sexual or physical abuse, or ongoing stress can increase the risk of developing GAD.

- **Medical conditions**: Certain medical conditions, such as heart disease, diabetes, or thyroid problems, can increase the risk of GAD.
- **Substance abuse**: Using drugs or alcohol can increase the risk of GAD, especially if the individual has a history of substance abuse.
- **Gender**: Women are more likely to develop GAD than men.
- **Age**: GAD can occur at any age, but it typically develops in childhood or adolescence.
- **Personality**: People with certain personality traits such as being perfectionist, pessimistic or introverted may be more prone to develop GAD.
- **Social and economic factors**: People who experience poverty, unemployment, or lack of social support may be more likely to develop GAD

It's important to note that having one or more risk factors does not mean that a person will definitely develop GAD. Many people with risk factors never develop the disorder, and many people who develop GAD have no known risk factors.

GAD can be treated, and most treatments include a mix of therapy, medications, and things you can do on your own. Cognitive-behavioral therapy (CBT) is an effective form of therapy for GAD. It helps people learn to identify and change negative thought patterns and behaviors that contribute to anxiety. Medications such as antidepressants and anti-anxiety medications may also be used to manage symptoms.

2. Panic Disorder

Panic disorder is a type of anxiety disorder characterized by recurrent, unexpected panic attacks. A panic attack is a sudden, intense feeling of fear or discomfort that can cause physical symptoms like a fast heartbeat, sweating, shaking, and trouble breathing. Panic attacks can happen at any time, even during sleep, and they can be so severe that they may be mistaken for a heart attack.

People with panic disorder may also feel anxious about having a panic attack in the future. This is called anticipatory anxiety. This can cause the person to stay away from places or situations that remind them of their panic attacks.

Symptoms

Symptoms of panic disorder typically include:

- Recurrent, unexpected panic attacks
- Persistent fear or worry about having another panic attack
- Avoidance of places or situations that may trigger panic attacks
- Physical symptoms such as rapid heartbeat, sweating, shaking, and difficulty breathing
- Fear or worry about the physical symptoms of a panic attack
- Fear or worry about losing control or going crazy
- Fear or worry about dying

Causes

No one knows for sure what causes panic disorder, but it is thought to be caused by a mix of genetic, environmental, and mental factors. Panic disorder is often linked to other mental health problems, like depression, generalized anxiety disorder, and drug abuse.

Risk Factors

Panic disorder is a complicated illness that can be caused by a mix of genetic, environmental, and mental factors. Some of the risk factors associated with panic disorder include:

- **Genetics**: There is some evidence to suggest that panic disorder may run in families, and that certain genetic variations may increase the risk of developing the disorder.
- **Trauma or stress:** Being in a traumatic situation, like a natural disaster, war, sexual or physical abuse, or being under

a lot of stress, can make it more likely that someone will develop panic disorder.

- **Medical conditions**: Certain medical conditions, such as heart disease, diabetes, or thyroid problems, can increase the risk of panic disorder.
- **Substance abuse**: Using drugs or alcohol can increase the risk of panic disorder, especially if the individual has a history of substance abuse.
- **Personality**: People with certain personality traits such as being perfectionist, pessimistic or introverted may be more prone to develop panic disorder.
- **Social and economic factors**: People who experience poverty, unemployment, or lack of social support may be more likely to develop panic disorder
- **Life events**: Some major life events such as marriage, divorce, childbirth, or job loss can also increase the risk of developing panic disorder

It's important to note that having one or more risk factors does not mean that a person will definitely develop panic disorder. Many people with risk factors never develop the disorder, and many people who develop panic disorder have no known risk factors.

Panic disorder can be treated, and most treatments include a mix of therapy, medications, and things you can do on your own. Cognitive-behavioral therapy (CBT) is an effective form of therapy for panic disorder that helps people learn to identify and change negative thought patterns and behaviors that contribute to anxiety. Medications such as antidepressants and anti-anxiety medications may also be used to manage symptoms.

3. Social Anxiety Disorder (SAD)

Social Anxiety Disorder (SAD), also known as social phobia, is a type of anxiety disorder characterized by excessive self-consciousness and fear of social situations. People with SAD feel very afraid or embarrassed in social situations and worry that others will judge them or reject them. In social situations, they may also have physical signs like blushing, sweating, or shaking. This kind of intense fear and anxiety can cause people to avoid certain social situations or go through them with a lot of pain.

SAD can show up in many ways, like being afraid to speak in public, eat or drink in public, use public restrooms, or even go on a date. The symptoms of SAD can have a big impact on daily life, making it hard for people to keep up with their relationships, do their jobs, or finish their education.

Symptoms

- Fear of being judged adversely in situations.
- Concern yourself with embarrassing or degrading yourself.
- Fear of interacting or conversing with strangers.
- Fear that people may see your anxiety.
- Fear of embarrassing bodily symptoms such as blushing, sweating, trembling, or having a wobbly voice.
- Fear of embarrassment causes people to avoid doing tasks or speaking to others.
- Avoid circumstances in which you may be the center of attention.
- Anxiety caused by a feared action or event.
- Anxiety or apprehension during social circumstances.
- After a social situation, analyze your performance and identify shortcomings in your interactions.
- The expectation of the worst possible outcomes after a poor social experience.

Causes

No one knows for sure what causes SAD, but it is thought that a mix of genetic, environmental, and psychological factors are to blame. Social Anxiety Disorder is also commonly found with other mental health conditions such as depression, generalized anxiety disorder, and substance abuse.

Risk Factors

Social Anxiety Disorder (SAD) can be influenced by a combination of genetic, environmental, and psychological factors. Some of the risk factors associated with SAD include:

- **Genetics**: There is some evidence to suggest that SAD may run in families, and that certain genetic variations may increase the risk of developing the disorder.
- **Trauma or stress**: Trauma, such as experiencing bullying, or ongoing stress can increase the risk of developing SAD.
- **Medical conditions**: Certain medical conditions, such as heart disease, diabetes, or thyroid problems, can increase the risk of SAD.
- **Substance abuse**: Using drugs or alcohol can increase the risk of SAD, especially if the individual has a history of substance abuse.
- **Personality**: People with certain personality traits such as being perfectionist, pessimistic or introverted may be more prone to develop SAD.
- **Social and economic factors**: People who experience poverty, unemployment, or lack of social support may be more likely to develop SAD
- **Life events**: Some major life events such as marriage, divorce, childbirth, or job loss can also increase the risk of developing SAD
- **Social skills**: People with poor social skills or lack of social support may be more prone to develop SAD

SAD can be treated, and most treatments include a mix of therapy, medications, and things you can do on your own. Cognitive-behavioral therapy (CBT) is an effective form of therapy for SAD. It helps people learn to identify and change negative thought patterns and behaviors that contribute to anxiety. Medications such as antidepressants and anti-anxiety medications may also be used to manage symptoms.

4. Phobias

A phobia is a type of anxiety disorder that causes people to be overly afraid of certain things or situations. Phobias are strong, long-lasting, and often crippling fears that can cause a lot of stress and get in the way of daily life. People with phobias may feel intense fear or panic when they encounter the thing or situation they fear, and they may go to great lengths to avoid it.

Some common phobias include:

- Agoraphobia: fear of open or public spaces
- Acrophobia: fear of heights
- Arachnophobia: fear of spiders
- Ophidiophobia: fear of snakes
- Cynophobia: fear of dogs
- Astraphobia: fear of thunder and lightning
- Aerophobia: fear of flying
- Emetophobia: fear of vomiting
- Mysophobia: fear of germs or dirt

Causes

Phobias can happen at any age and are usually caused by a mix of genetic, environmental, and mental factors. A traumatic event or a history of abuse can also make it more likely that someone will develop a phobia.

Risk Factors

Phobias are a type of anxiety disorder that can be caused by a mix of genes, the environment, and the way a person thinks and feels. Some of the risk factors associated with phobias include:

- **Genes**: There is some evidence that phobias may run in families and that some genetic differences may make it more likely that someone will have a phobia.
- **Trauma or stress**: Having a phobia is more likely if you have been through a traumatic event or have a history of being abused.
- **Medical conditions**: Certain medical conditions, such as heart disease, diabetes, or thyroid problems, can increase the risk of phobias.
- **Substance abuse**: Using drugs or alcohol can increase the risk of phobias, especially if the individual has a history of substance abuse.
- **Personality**: People with certain personality traits such as being perfectionist, pessimistic or introverted may be more prone to develop phobias.
- **Social and economic factors**: People who experience poverty, unemployment, or lack of social support may be more likely to develop phobias
- **Life events**: Some major life events such as marriage, divorce, childbirth, or job loss can also increase the risk of developing phobias
- **Social skills**: People with poor social skills or lack of social support may be more prone to develop phobias
- **Past experiences**: people who experienced a traumatic event or a near-death experience might develop a phobia related to that situation or object.

It's important to note that having one or more risk factors does not mean that a person will definitely develop a phobia. Many people with risk factors never develop the disorder, and many people who develop phobias have no known risk factors.

Phobias can be treated, and most treatments include a mix of therapy, medication, and things you can do on your own. Cognitive-behavioral therapy (CBT) is an effective form of therapy for phobias. It helps people learn to identify and change negative thought patterns and behaviors that contribute to anxiety. Medications such as antidepressants and anti-anxiety medications may also be used to manage symptoms.

5. Obsessive Compulsive Disorder (OCD)

Obsessive-Compulsive Disorder (OCD) is a type of anxiety disorder that is marked by persistent, uncontrollable thoughts, urges, or images (obsessions) and repetitive behaviors or mental acts (compulsions) that the person feels driven to do.

People with OCD may have obsessions, which are unwanted, repeated thoughts, images, or urges that are hard to control or ignore. These obsessions can cause significant anxiety, fear, or disgust. In order to try to get rid of this anxiety, people with OCD may do things over and over again (compulsions) like cleaning, counting, checking, or praying a lot.

Symptoms

Symptoms of OCD typically include:

- Persistent, unwanted thoughts, images, or impulses (obsessions)
- Repetitive behaviors or mental acts (compulsions)
- Difficulty controlling or reducing the obsessions or compulsions
- Significant distress or impairment in daily life

Examples of common obsessions and compulsions include:

- Fear of contamination and excessive cleaning
- Fear of harm and excessive checking
- Obsessions with symmetry and exactness, leading to arranging and ordering compulsions
- Harmful thoughts about oneself or others and compulsive praying or mental acts to neutralize or counteract them.

Causes

The exact cause of OCD is not known, but it is thought to be related to a combination of genetic, environmental, and psychological factors. OCD is also often found in people who have other mental health problems, like depression, generalized anxiety disorder, or drug abuse.

Risk Factors

Obsessive-Compulsive Disorder (OCD) is a complicated condition that can be caused by a mix of genetic, environmental, and psychological factors. Some of the risk factors associated with OCD include:

- **Genetics**: There is some evidence to suggest that OCD may run in families, and that certain genetic variations may increase the risk of developing the disorder.
- **Trauma or stress**: Trauma, such as experiencing a natural disaster, combat, or sexual or physical abuse, or ongoing stress can increase the risk of developing OCD.
- **Medical conditions**: Certain medical conditions, such as heart disease, diabetes, or thyroid problems, can increase the risk of OCD.
- **Substance abuse**: Using drugs or alcohol can increase the risk of OCD, especially if the individual has a history of substance abuse.
- **Gender**: Women are more likely to develop OCD than men.
- **Age**: OCD can occur at any age, but it typically develops in childhood or adolescence.
- **Personality**: People with certain personality traits such as being perfectionist, pessimistic or introverted may be more prone to develop OCD.
- **Social and economic factors**: People who experience poverty, unemployment, or lack of social support may be more likely to develop OCD

- **Brain function and structure**: Research has shown that certain areas of the brain and their functions are linked to OCD symptoms.

It's important to note that having one or more risk factors does not mean that a person will definitely develop OCD. Many people with risk factors never develop the disorder, and many people who develop OCD have no known risk factors.

OCD can be treated, and most treatments include a mix of therapy, medications, and ways to help yourself. Cognitive-behavioral therapy (CBT) is an effective form of therapy for OCD that helps people learn to identify and change negative thought patterns and behaviors that contribute to anxiety. Medications such as antidepressants and anti-anxiety medications may also be used to manage symptoms.

6. Post-Traumatic Stress Disorder

Post-Traumatic Stress Disorder (PTSD) is a mental health condition that can happen after a person goes through or sees a traumatic event, like a natural disaster, war, sexual or physical assault, or a serious accident. PTSD is characterized by a range of symptoms that can include:

- Intrusive, distressing memories, nightmares, or flashbacks of the traumatic event
- Avoidance behaviors, such as avoiding people, places, or activities that may trigger memories of the trauma
- Negative changes in mood and cognition, such as feeling detached or emotionally numb, having difficulty feeling positive emotions, or having difficulty remembering key aspects of the trauma
- Hyperarousal symptoms, such as feeling irritable, easily startled, or having difficulty sleeping or concentrating

PTSD can have a significant impact on a person's life, making it difficult for them to function in their daily lives. People with PTSD may experience difficulties with relationships, have trouble at work or school, and have problems with substance abuse.

Causes

It's not completely clear what causes PTSD, but it's thought to be a mix of genetic, environmental, and psychological factors. PTSD is often linked to other mental health problems, like depression, generalized anxiety disorder, and drug abuse.

Risk Factors

Post-Traumatic Stress Disorder (PTSD) can be caused by a mix of psychological, genetic, and environmental factors. Some of the risk factors associated with PTSD include:

- **Trauma**: Experiencing or witnessing a traumatic event, such as combat, sexual or physical assault, a serious accident, or natural disasters, is the most significant risk factor for developing PTSD.
- **Severity and duration of the trauma**: The more severe and prolonged the trauma is, the more likely a person is to develop PTSD
- **Proximity to the traumatic event**: People who were physically close to the traumatic event and directly impacted by it are at a higher risk of developing PTSD
- **Pre-existing mental health conditions**: People with pre-existing mental health conditions, such as depression or anxiety, are at a higher risk of developing PTSD
- **Lack of social support**: People who have little or no social support are at a higher risk of developing PTSD
- **Genetics**: There is some evidence to suggest that certain genetic variations may increase the risk of developing PTSD
- **Gender**: Women are more likely to develop PTSD than men
- **Age**: Children and older adults are more at risk of developing PTSD

- **Substance abuse**: People who have a history of substance abuse are at a higher risk of developing PTSD

It's important to note that having one or more risk factors does not mean that a person will definitely develop PTSD. Many people with risk factors never develop the disorder, and many people who develop PTSD have no known risk factors.

PTSD can be treated, and most treatments include a mix of therapy, medications, and things you can do on your own. Cognitive-behavioral therapy (CBT) is an effective form of therapy for PTSD that helps people learn to identify and change negative thought patterns and behaviors that contribute to anxiety. Medications such as antidepressants and anti-anxiety medications may also be used to manage symptoms.

7. Separation Anxiety Disorder

Separation Anxiety Disorder (SAD) is a type of anxiety disorder characterized by excessive and persistent fear or distress related to separation from home or from loved ones. Most children and teens are diagnosed with SAD, but it can also happen to adults.

Symptoms

Symptoms of SAD typically include:

- Persistent and excessive fear or distress when separated from home or loved ones
- Refusal to go to school, work, or other places or events because of fear of separation
- Recurrent nightmares or night terrors related to separation
- Physical symptoms such as headaches, stomachaches, or nausea when faced with separation
- Difficulty sleeping alone or away from loved ones
- Persistent thoughts or worries about harm coming to loved ones

Causes

No one knows for sure what causes SAD, but it is thought to be a mix of genetic, environmental, and psychological factors. SAD is also often linked to other mental health problems, like depression, generalized anxiety disorder, and drug abuse.

Risk Factors

Separation Anxiety Disorder (SAD) can be influenced by a combination of genetic, environmental, and psychological factors. Some of the risk factors associated with SAD include:

- **Genetics**: Some evidence suggests that SAD may run in families and that some genetic differences may make it more likely that someone will get the disorder.
- **Trauma or stress**: Trauma, such as experiencing a separation or loss of a loved one, or ongoing stress can increase the risk of developing SAD.
- **Medical conditions**: Certain medical conditions, such as heart disease, diabetes, or thyroid problems, can increase the risk of SAD.
- **Substance abuse**: Using drugs or alcohol can increase the risk of SAD, especially if the individual has a history of substance abuse.
- **Age**: SAD is most commonly diagnosed in children and adolescents, but it can also occur in adults.
- **Personality**: People with certain personality traits such as being perfectionist, pessimistic or introverted may be more prone to develop SAD.
- **Social and economic factors**: People who experience poverty, unemployment, or lack of social support may be more likely to develop SAD
- **Life events**: Some major life events such as marriage, divorce, childbirth, or job loss can also increase the risk of developing SAD

- **Social skills**: People with poor social skills or lack of social support may be more prone to develop SAD

It's important to note that having one or more risk factors does not mean that a person will definitely develop SAD. Many people with risk factors never develop the disorder, and many people who develop SAD have no known risk factors.

SAD can be treated, and most treatments include a mix of therapy, medications, and things you can do on your own. Cognitive-behavioral therapy (CBT) is an effective form of therapy for SAD. It helps people learn to identify and change negative thought patterns and behaviors that contribute to anxiety. Medications such as antidepressants and anti-anxiety medications may also be used to manage symptoms.

8. Selective Mutism

Selective Mutism (SM) is a type of anxiety disorder characterized by an individual's inability to speak in certain social situations, such as at school, work, or in public places, despite being able to speak in other settings, such as at home with family members. Selective Mutism is a complex condition that can have a significant impact on a person's daily life.

Symptoms

Symptoms of SM typically include:

- Persistent inability to speak in certain social situations, such as at school or work, despite being able to speak in other settings
- Difficulty initiating or maintaining conversation in social situations
- Extreme shyness or social anxiety in social situations
- Difficulty making eye contact or nonverbal communication in social situations

- Physical symptoms such as sweating, shaking or blushing when faced with social situations

Causes

No one knows for sure what causes SM, but it is thought to be a mix of genetic, environmental, and psychological factors. SM is also often found in people who have other mental health problems, like depression, generalized anxiety disorder, and drug abuse.

Risk Factors

Selective Mutism (SM) can be influenced by a combination of genetic, environmental, and psychological factors. Some of the risk factors associated with SM include:

- **Genetics**: Some evidence suggests that SM may run in families and that some genetic differences may make it more likely to get the disorder.
- **Trauma or stress**: Trauma, such as experiencing a separation or loss of a loved one, or ongoing stress can increase the risk of developing SM.
- **Medical conditions**: Certain medical conditions, such as heart disease, diabetes, or thyroid problems, can increase the risk of SM.
- **Substance abuse**: Using drugs or alcohol can increase the risk of SM, especially if the individual has a history of substance abuse.
- **Age**: SM is most commonly diagnosed in children and adolescents, but it can also occur in adults.
- **Personality**: People with certain personality traits such as being perfectionist, pessimistic or introverted may be more prone to develop SM.
- **Social and economic factors**: People who experience poverty, unemployment, or lack of social support may be more likely to develop SM

- **Life events**: Some major life events such as marriage, divorce, childbirth, or job loss can also increase the risk of developing SM
- **Social skills**: People with poor social skills or lack of social support may be more prone to develop SM
- **Family dynamics**: Children who come from families with a history of anxiety, shyness, or perfectionism are more at risk of developing SM

It's important to note that having one or more risk factors does not mean that a person will definitely develop SM. Many people with risk factors never develop the disorder, and many people who develop SM have no known risk factors.

SM can be treated, and most treatments involve a mix of therapy, medication, and self-help methods. Behavioral therapy is an effective form of therapy for SM because it helps people learn to identify and change negative thought patterns and behaviors that contribute to anxiety. Medications such as antidepressants and anti-anxiety medications may also be used to manage symptoms.

9. Body Dysmorphic Disorder

Body Dysmorphic Disorder (BDD) is a type of mental disorder characterized by a preoccupation with one or more perceived flaws or defects in one's physical appearance that are not observable or appear slight to others. This preoccupation causes significant distress and interferes with daily functioning.

People with BDD think and act in ways that are out of their control and do things like over-grooming, getting cosmetic procedures, or looking for reassurance about how they look. Because they care so much about how they look, they may also avoid social situations, work, and school.

Symptoms

Symptoms of BDD typically include:

- Preoccupation with one or more perceived flaws or defects in one's physical appearance, which are not observable or appear slight to others
- Constant comparison of one's appearance to others
- Repetitive behaviors such as checking, grooming, or seeking reassurance about one's appearance
- Avoiding social situations, work, and school due to preoccupation with one's appearance
- Engaging in excessive grooming, such as hair plucking, skin picking, or excessive use of makeup
- Seeking unnecessary cosmetic procedures to improve perceived flaws
- Having low self-esteem and self-worth as a result of preoccupation with one's appearance
- Having co-occurring disorders such as anxiety, depression, and obsessive-compulsive disorder (OCD)

Causes

BDD is not fully understood, but it is thought that it is caused by a mix of genetic, environmental, and mental factors. Research suggests that BDD may be caused by changes in the structure and function of the brain, especially in parts of the brain that deal with body image and perception.

Risk Factors

Body Dysmorphic Disorder (BDD) can be caused by a mix of environmental, genetic, and mental factors. Some of the risk factors associated with BDD include:

- **Genetics**: There is some evidence to suggest that BDD may run in families, and that certain genetic variations may increase the risk of developing the disorder.

- **Trauma or stress**: Trauma, such as experiencing bullying, abuse, or neglect, or ongoing stress can increase the risk of developing BDD.
- **Medical conditions**: Certain medical conditions, such as heart disease, diabetes, or thyroid problems, can increase the risk of BDD.
- **Substance abuse**: Using drugs or alcohol can increase the risk of BDD, especially if the individual has a history of substance abuse.
- **Age**: BDD is more commonly diagnosed in adolescents and young adults, but it can also occur in children and older adults.
- **Personality**: People with certain personality traits such as being perfectionist, pessimistic or introverted may be more prone to develop BDD.
- **Social and economic factors**: People who experience poverty, unemployment, or lack of social support may be more likely to develop BDD
- **Life events**: Some major life events, such as marriage, divorce, childbirth, or job loss, can also increase the risk of developing BDD.
- **Social skills**: People with poor social skills or lack of social support may be more prone to develop BDD
- **Exposure to media**: Exposure to idealized images of beauty in the media can increase the risk of developing BDD

It's important to note that having one or more risk factors does not mean that a person will definitely develop BDD. Many people with risk factors never develop the disorder, and many people who develop BDD have no known risk factors.

BDD can be treated, and most treatments involve a mix of therapy, medication, and self-help methods. Cognitive-behavioral therapy (CBT) is an effective form of therapy for BDD, which helps people learn to identify and change negative thought patterns and behaviors that contribute to anxiety. Medications such as antidepressants and anti-anxiety medications may also be used to manage symptoms.

10. Illness Anxiety Disorder (Hypochondria)

Illness Anxiety Disorder (IAD), also known as Hypochondriasis, is a type of anxiety disorder characterized by excessive and persistent preoccupation with the fear of having a serious illness, despite having no or only mild symptoms. People with IAD are always worried that they have a serious disease, which causes a lot of stress and makes it hard to go about their daily lives.

Symptoms

Symptoms of IAD typically include:

- Persistent and excessive preoccupation with the fear of having a serious illness
- Constant self-examination and monitoring of bodily symptoms
- Repeatedly seeking medical attention and reassurance for mild or imagined symptoms
- Difficulty accepting medical reassurance that no serious illness is present
- Avoiding certain situations or activities due to fear of illness
- Having low self-esteem and self-worth as a result of preoccupation with illness
- Having co-occurring disorders such as depression, anxiety, and obsessive-compulsive disorder (OCD)

Causes

No one knows for sure what causes IAD, but it is thought to be a mix of genetic, environmental, and psychological factors. Research suggests that IAD may be caused by changes in the structure and function of the brain, especially in areas that deal with how the body feels.

Risk Factors

Illness Anxiety Disorder (IAD) can be influenced by a combination of genetic, environmental, and psychological factors. Some of the risk factors associated with IAD include:

- **Genetics**: There is some evidence to suggest that IAD may run in families, and that certain genetic variations may increase the risk of developing the disorder.
- **Trauma or stress**: Trauma, such as experiencing a serious illness or the loss of a loved one, or ongoing stress can increase the risk of developing IAD.
- **Medical conditions**: Certain medical conditions, such as chronic pain or autoimmune disorders, can increase the risk of IAD.
- **Substance abuse**: Using drugs or alcohol can increase the risk of IAD, especially if the individual has a history of substance abuse.
- **Age**: IAD can occur at any age but is more commonly diagnosed in adults.
- **Personality**: People with certain personality traits, such as being perfectionist, pessimistic, or introverted, may be more prone to developing IAD.
- **Social and economic factors**: People who experience poverty, unemployment, or lack of social support may be more likely to develop IAD
- **Life events**: Some major life events such as marriage, divorce, childbirth, or job loss can also increase the risk of developing IAD
- **Social skills**: People with poor social skills or lack of social support may be more prone to develop IAD
- **History of health anxiety**: Individuals who have had a history of health anxiety in the past are at a higher risk of developing IAD.

It's important to note that having one or more risk factors does not mean that a person will definitely develop IAD. Many people with risk factors never develop the disorder, and many people who develop IAD have no known risk factors.

IAD can be treated, and most treatments involve a mix of therapy, medications, and things you can do on your own. Cognitive-behavioral therapy (CBT) is an effective form of therapy for IAD, which helps people learn to identify and change negative thought patterns and behaviors that contribute to anxiety. Medications such as antidepressants and anti-anxiety medications may also be used to manage symptoms.

UNDERSTANDING THE BASICS OF MINDFULNESS AND ITS BENEFITS FOR MANAGING ANXIETY

Mindfulness is the practice of being present in the moment and paying attention to one's thoughts, feelings, and physical sensations in a non-judgmental and accepting way. It is a technique that has been studied a lot and shown to help people deal with anxiety.

People who practice mindfulness are taught to pay attention to the present rather than thinking about the past or worrying about the future. This can help to reduce the amount of time that people spend ruminating on negative thoughts and worries, which can be a major contributor to anxiety. Mindfulness also makes people more aware of their thoughts and feelings, which can help them understand their anxiety better and come up with ways to deal with it.

The benefits of mindfulness for managing anxiety include:

1. **Decreased symptoms of anxiety**: Regular practice of mindfulness has been found to decrease symptoms of anxiety, such as worry, rumination, and physical symptoms such as muscle tension.
2. **Increased ability to regulate emotions**: Mindfulness can help individuals to become more aware of their emotions and develop strategies for managing them, which can be particularly helpful for those with anxiety disorders.
3. **Improved focus and concentration**: Mindfulness can help individuals to focus on the present moment, which can improve concentration and focus, making it easier to complete tasks and make decisions.
4. **Better sleep**: Mindfulness can help to reduce the amount of time that people spend worrying, which can improve sleep quality and help individuals feel more rested and refreshed.

5. **Improved relationships:** Mindfulness can help people improve their relationships and communication by making them more present and sensitive to others.

Mindfulness is not a replacement for professional treatment, but it can be used as a complementary therapy in the treatment of anxiety and other mental health conditions. Mindfulness can be taught in classes, through books, online, or with the help of a trained therapist.

Mindfulness Meditation Techniques And How To Practice Them Effectively

Mindfulness and relaxation techniques are forms of alternative treatment for anxiety disorders. The goal of these techniques is to teach the person to be in the present moment and to notice their thoughts, feelings, and physical sensations without judging them. Mindfulness and relaxation techniques can help people deal with anxiety by reducing stress and tension and giving them a sense of calm and well-being.

Introduction To Mindfulness And Its Benefits For Managing Anxiety

It is all too easy to speed through life without pausing to take it all in.

Paying more attention to the present moment—to your own thoughts and feelings as well as to the world around you—can help you feel better mentally.

This awareness is sometimes referred to as "mindfulness" by others. Mindfulness can help us appreciate life more fully and better understand ourselves. You can work on developing it in your own life.

What Exactly Is Mindfulness

Mindfulness means paying attention to what is going on inside and outside of us right now.

It's easy to lose sight of the world around us. It's also easy to lose touch with how our bodies are feeling and wind up living "in our heads," caught up in our thoughts without pausing to consider how those thoughts are influencing our emotions and behavior.

Reconnecting with our body and the sensations it produces is an important aspect of mindfulness. This entails focusing on the sights, sounds, scents, and tastes of the present moment. It could be as basic as the feel of a banister as we walk upstairs.

Being aware of our thoughts and feelings as they happen in the present moment is another important part of being mindful.

How Mindfulness Improves Mental Health

When it comes to anxiety disorders, mindfulness and relaxation techniques can help individuals to:

- Decrease worry and rumination by shifting the focus away from negative thoughts and emotions
- Increase self-awareness, which can help individuals to identify the triggers of their anxiety and develop coping strategies
- Improve emotional regulation, by helping individuals to manage their emotions in a healthy way
- Increase resilience and adaptability, by teaching individuals to be more flexible and open to change
- Increase self-compassion, by encouraging individuals to be kind and understanding towards themselves
- Improve sleep quality, by reducing stress and tension

Examples of mindfulness and relaxation techniques that can be used to manage anxiety disorders include mindfulness meditation, yoga, tai chi, progressive muscle relaxation, guided imagery, aromatherapy, and biofeedback. These techniques can be used alone or in combination with other forms of treatment, such as therapy or medication. It's important to work with a mental health professional to figure out the best way to help a specific person.

Increasing our awareness of the present moment can help us enjoy the world around us more and better understand ourselves.

When we become more aware of the present moment, we begin to re-experience things we previously took for granted.

Mindfulness also helps us become more aware of the flow of our thoughts and feelings and how we can get caught up in that flow in ways that aren't helpful.

This allows us to step back from our thoughts and recognize their patterns. We can gradually train ourselves to recognize when our ideas take over and recognize that thoughts are only "mental happenings" that do not have to rule us.

Mindfulness can assist us in dealing with problems more effectively. "Am I attempting to fix this by ruminating about it, or am I just getting caught up in my thoughts?" we can ask.

This kind of awareness could also help us notice signs of stress or worry sooner and deal with them better.

The National Institute for Health and Care Excellence (NICE) says that mindfulness-based therapy is a good way to treat depression that isn't too bad.

NICE also suggests that organizations make mindfulness available to all employees to improve mental health at work.

How To Be More Mindful

The first step toward mindfulness is to remind yourself to pay attention to your thoughts, feelings, physical sensations, and the world around you.

1. Take Note Of The Mundane.

We can notice the feelings of things as we go about our daily lives, such as the food we consume and the air moving past our bodies as we walk.

2. Maintain A Consistent Schedule.

It can be beneficial to choose a regular time, such as your commute to work or a lunchtime walk, during which you decide to be aware of the sensations caused by the world around you.

3. Experiment With Something New.

Trying new things, such as sitting in a different seat in meetings or going to a new restaurant for lunch, can also help you notice the world in a fresh light.

4. Keep An Eye On Your Thoughts.

Mindfulness might be difficult for some people to practice. When they stop what they're doing, a flood of thoughts and fears descend on them.

It's important to remember that mindfulness isn't about making these thoughts disappear; rather, it's about perceiving them as mental events that come and go. This can be difficult at first, but it is attainable with patience and persistence.

Some folks find that doing mild yoga or walking helps them cope with an overly active mind.

5. Describe Your Thoughts And Feelings

To build awareness of thoughts and feelings, some people find it beneficial to silently label them: "Here's the thought that I might flunk that exam" or "This is anxiety."

6. Break Free From The Past And The Future

You can practice mindfulness anywhere, but it can be especially helpful when you realize you've been thinking about past problems or worrying about things that might bother you in the future for a long time.

Various Mindfulness Practices

Along with practicing mindfulness in everyday life, it can be helpful to set aside time for a more formal mindfulness practice.

Mindfulness meditation involves sitting still and paying attention to thoughts, sounds, the way you feel when you breathe, or parts of your body. When your mind wanders, you bring it back.

But for this book, we would be looking at the following mindfulness techniques, in our quest to curbing anxiety disorders

1. Yoga Technique
2. Diaphragmatic Breathing Technique
3. Progressive Muscle Relaxation Technique
4. Guided Imagery And Visualization
5. The Use Of Aromatherapy And Essential Oils
6. Mindful Self-Compassion
7. Mindful Movement
8. Mindful-Based Stress Reduction (MBSR)
9. Acupuncture

Yoga And Mindfulness: How To Use Yoga Poses And Breathing Exercises To Reduce Anxiety

Due to its physical and emotional benefits, yoga's popularity continues to increase. Practicing yoga on your own can help you avoid and deal with stress, which is a common goal for people who want to grow in a positive way and work on improving themselves.

A yoga routine may include breathing, meditation, and relaxation, thereby relieving emotional stress. They also increase the release of mood-boosting endorphins, which are the feel-good hormones that can have a favorable effect on how you deal with stress.

During your yoga practice, focusing on the present moment makes you more aware, helps you focus better, and calms your mind.

As you become more aware that your body sensations, thoughts, and emotions don't last forever, it may be easier to let go of your attachments to good, bad, and neutral experiences. You may also discover how to foster emotions such as love, pleasure, and tranquility.

What Does Research Say About Yoga For Stress Relief?

Yoga's stress-relieving effects are supported by abundant scientific evidence.

Hatha yoga done three times per week for four weeks has a favorable effect on women, according to a 2018 study. Significant reductions in stress, depression, and anxiety were observed after 12 sessions.

Based on these results, it seems that yoga can be used as a therapy supplement and may reduce the need for prescription drugs. More research needs to be done to find out what role yoga plays in the long-term treatment of stress, depression, and anxiety.

Yoga stretches reduce cortisol levels and increase parasympathetic nerve activity, which promotes relaxation, according to a small study conducted on adult men in 2020.

In a 2020 study, it was shown that persons who practiced yoga nidra meditation for 11 minutes per day for 30 days experienced a reduction in stress, an improvement in their overall health, and an improvement in the quality of their sleep.

Yoga nidra practice also increased mindfulness and diminished negative emotions. After six weeks, these advantages remained unchanged.

How To Reduce Stress Using Yoga Breathing

Breathing exercises, known in Sanskrit as "Pranayama," teach you to relax, control your breathing, and breathe deeply. This reduces stress and calms the mind and body. Breathing exercises can also improve sleep quality and foster mindfulness.

When you want to focus on relaxation during the day or when you are performing yoga, you can perform breathing exercises. These methods also work when you are feeling bad or when things are hard.

A lot of people turn to yoga when they start to feel anxious or under a lot of stress. You may discover that concentrating on both your breath and your ability to be present in each position will help quiet negative thought chatter and improve your mood overall.

It is essential to meet yourself where you are. If you are open to the practice, practicing one or two postures for just a few minutes every day can have a significant effect.

To get the most out of your yoga session, pay attention to how you feel as you move from one pose to the next. Permit yourself to feel and experience all of your emotions.

If your mind starts to wander, bring it gently back to the mat and keep practicing.

Yoga Poses That Can Help Curb Anxiety

There are several types of yoga poses that can help curb anxiety disorders. Some of the most commonly recommended poses are (we won't include pictures in this book because you can find them for free on the internet or in yoga classes):

A. Child's Pose (Balasana)

This pose helps to calm the mind and relax the body, making it a great option for those dealing with anxiety.

Child's pose, also known as *"Balasana"* in Sanskrit, is a restorative yoga pose that can help to calm the mind and reduce symptoms of anxiety. This pose involves sitting on the heels with the knees wide apart and the forehead resting on the floor. The arms can be stretched out in front or relaxed by the side of the body. The pose can help release tension in the back, shoulders, and neck, which are common areas of tension for people experiencing anxiety. Additionally, the position of the head and the focus on deep, slow breathing can help to bring a sense of calm and grounding to the mind. Some practitioners also find that the position of the head and the sensation of the forehead resting on the ground can help to release feelings of stress and worry.

B. Downward-Facing Dog (Adho Mukha Svanasana)

This pose helps reduce stress and tension in the body, making it a great option for those dealing with anxiety.

The downward-facing dog yoga pose, which is also called "Adho Mukha Svanasana," can help people with anxiety disorders because it is a calming, grounding pose that helps the body release tension. This pose can help reduce stress and anxiety by calming the nervous system and giving you a sense of balance and well-being. The pose is often used as a way to release anxiety and tension in the body. This is a great yoga pose for those who are feeling anxious, stressed, or overwhelmed. It can help to release tension and promote a sense of calm and serenity. It can also help people focus and concentrate better and feel less worried, scared, and restless.

C. Warrior II (Virabhadrasana II)

This pose helps to increase self-confidence and self-esteem, which can be beneficial for those dealing with anxiety.

Warrior 2 yoga pose, also called "Virabhadrasana II," is thought to help people with anxiety disorders feel stronger and more stable. This pose involves standing with the feet wide apart and then turning one foot out and the other foot in. The arms are then extended out to the sides, with one arm facing forward and the other arm facing back. This creates a sense of grounding and balance in the body, which can help calm the mind and reduce feelings of anxiety. The pose also encourages deep breathing, which can help calm the body and reduce stress. Overall, the Warrior 2 yoga pose can help to create a sense of inner peace and calm, which can be beneficial for managing symptoms of anxiety disorders.

D. Eagle Pose (Garudasana)

This pose helps to improve balance and concentration, which can be beneficial for those dealing with anxiety.

Eagle pose, or *"Garudasana"* in Sanskrit, is a standing balance pose that requires focus and concentration. This pose can help people with anxiety disorders because it helps the body feel grounded and stable, which can calm the mind. The grounding effect of the pose can also help reduce feelings of worry and stress and promote feelings of stability and balance. Also, eagle pose can help improve the strength and flexibility of the legs and core, which can lead to better posture and a healthier body overall. This pose is also thought to stimulate the nervous system and can help to relieve tension in the shoulders and neck, which can be areas of the body that tend to hold tension when we are anxious.

E. Happy Baby Pose (Ananda Balasana):

This pose helps to release tension in the back and hips, making it a great option for those dealing with anxiety.

The Happy Baby yoga pose, also known as *"Ananda Balasana,"* can help to reduce anxiety by calming the mind and promoting relaxation. This pose involves lying on your back and drawing your knees into your chest while holding onto the outer edges of your feet. This position can help release tension in the lower back and hips, which can be areas where people tend to hold stress. Deep breathing, which is needed to do this pose, can also help relax the body and lessen feelings of anxiety. It also gently massages the internal organs and calms the brain, which helps release stress and anxiety at any time. It is a great way to relax the body and mind, and it can be done anytime, anywhere.

F. Cat-Cow Pose (Marjaryasana-Bitilasana):

This pose helps to release tension in the spine and neck, making it a great option for those dealing with anxiety.

The cat-cow yoga pose, also known as "Marjaryasana-Bitilasana," is a gentle flow between two poses that can help to release tension in the spine and neck. This flow can help to increase mobility in the spine and can be a helpful way to release tension and stress. By moving the head and spine in a circular motion, the cat-cow pose can help to release tension in the shoulders, neck, and lower back, which can help to reduce feelings of anxiety and stress. Focusing on your breathing during this pose can also help calm the mind and make you feel more relaxed. People with anxiety disorders can benefit from this yoga pose because it can help them become more flexible, let go of tension and stress, and feel more calm and relaxed.

G. Legs-Up-The-Wall (Viparita Karani):

This pose helps reduce stress and tension in the body, making it a great option for those dealing with anxiety.

Legs-Up-The-Wall pose, also known as *"Viparita Karani,"* is a restorative yoga pose that can help to calm the mind and reduce anxiety. This pose involves lying on your back and resting your legs up against a wall. The position of the legs and the angle of the hips create a gentle inversion, which can help calm the nervous system and reduce stress. Also, the pose requires you to pay attention to your breath and be in the moment, which can help you be more mindful and have fewer anxiety-related negative thoughts. This pose is also great for reducing fatigue, headaches, and stress. Additionally, this pose helps in relieving tension in the legs, lower back, and neck.

H. Corpse Pose (Savasana):

This pose helps to relax the body and calm the mind, making it a great option for those dealing with anxiety.

The corpse pose, also known as "Savasana," is a relaxation pose that can be helpful in curbing anxiety disorders. When practicing this pose, the individual lies on their back with their arms and legs extended and relaxed. The pose makes it easier to let go of physical and mental tension, so the person can let go of any worries or bad thoughts they may be holding on to. The pose also aids in slowing breathing and heart rate, which can have a calming effect on both the body and mind. Also, the pose can be used to help you pay attention to the present, which is an important part of practicing mindfulness. This can help people with anxiety disorders learn how to be more aware and focus on the here and now instead of worrying about the past or future.

It is best to talk to a professional yoga teacher about how to do these poses in a safe and effective way.

In addition to these yoga poses, you can spend ten to fifteen minutes per day practicing pranayama and meditation. Yoga is a great way to make your body more flexible, and it can even help you lose weight.

Mindful Breathing Exercises: How To Use Diaphragmatic Breathing To Reduce Anxiety

Diaphragmatic breathing, also known as belly breathing or deep breathing, is a technique that can help reduce anxiety by promoting a sense of calm and relaxation. In this type of breathing, the diaphragm, a muscle at the bottom of the lungs, is used to control the breath.

To practice diaphragmatic breathing, find a quiet and comfortable place to sit or lie down. Place one hand on your chest and the other on your belly. Take a slow, deep breath through your nose, allowing your belly to rise as you fill your lungs with air. Hold your breath for a moment, then exhale slowly through your mouth, allowing your belly to fall.

As you continue to breathe deeply and slowly, focus your attention on the sensation of the breath moving in and out of your body. Try to keep your chest still and let your breath move through your diaphragm.

You can also try counting your breaths or repeating a soothing word or phrase to yourself as you breathe. Repeat this for several minutes.

By focusing on your breath and keeping your mind in the present moment, diaphragmatic breathing can help reduce anxiety and promote relaxation. It can also help ease anxiety symptoms like racing thoughts, fast breathing, and muscle tension. Diaphragmatic breathing can be practiced anytime and anywhere, making it a great tool to have in your anxiety management toolbox.

Progressive Muscle Relaxation (PMS) Techniques: How To Use The Technique To Reduce Muscle Tension And Anxiety

Progressive muscle relaxation (PMR) is a technique that involves tensing and then relaxing different muscle groups in the body to reduce muscle tension and anxiety. The technique is based on the idea that muscle tension and anxiety go hand in hand and that anxiety can be reduced by reducing muscle tension.

To use PMR, one begins by finding a quiet and comfortable place to sit or lie down. Then, starting with the feet and working up to the head, one tightens and then relaxes each group of muscles in the body. The process typically takes around 20 to 30 minutes.

When tensing a muscle group, one should do so for around 5–10 seconds and then release the tension for around 20–30 seconds, focusing on the sensation of the muscle relaxing. As one moves through the different muscle groups, it is important to pay attention to the sensations in each muscle group and to release any tension that may still be present.

PMR can be an effective tool for reducing muscle tension and anxiety. It can be done daily and combined with other relaxation techniques, such as deep breathing and visualization. It can also be used as a coping strategy during times of stress or anxiety.

Guided Imagery And Visualization: How To Use Guided Imagery And Visualization To Manage Anxiety

Guided imagery and visualization are relaxation techniques that involve using the imagination to create mental images or scenarios that are calming and soothing. The goal of these techniques is to reduce anxiety by shifting one's focus away from negative thoughts and feelings and instead directing attention towards a more peaceful and relaxed state.

To use guided imagery and visualization to manage anxiety, one can begin by finding a quiet and comfortable place to sit or lie down. Next, close your eyes and focus on your breath, taking deep and slow inhales and exhales.

Begin to imagine a peaceful place or scenario that brings you calm and comfort. This could be a beach, a forest, a garden, or any other place that you find soothing. As you visualize this place, try to incorporate as many sensory details as possible, such as the sound of the waves, the smell of the flowers, the feel of the grass under your feet, etc.

As you continue to focus on this peaceful scene, imagine yourself becoming more and more relaxed. You may also want to add some positive self-talk or affirmations to this visualization, such as "I am calm and relaxed," "I am in control of my anxiety," and "I am safe."

It is important to practice this technique regularly, even when you are not feeling anxious, so that you can call upon it more easily during times of stress. With regular practice, guided imagery and visualization can become effective tools for managing anxiety.

The Use Of Aromatherapy And Essential Oils For Relaxation And Reducing Anxiety Symptoms

Aromatherapy is the use of essential oils from plants to help people feel better physically and emotionally. Essential oils are very concentrated extracts of plants that have been used for their healing properties for hundreds of years. When inhaled or applied topically, these oils can affect the body and mind in a variety of ways.

The use of essential oils for anxiety relief can be done through inhalation or topical application. Inhalation is the most common method of use and can be done by diffusing the oil in a room, adding a few drops to a warm bath, or inhaling the oil directly from the bottle. Topical application can be done by adding a few drops of the oil to a carrier oil and massaging it into the skin.

Lavender, chamomile, bergamot, ylang-ylang, and vetiver are all essential oils that are often used to calm anxiety. These oils have a calming effect on the nervous system and can help reduce feelings of tension and stress. They can also help improve sleep and promote feelings of relaxation.

It's important to remember that you should use essential oils with care and with the help of a medical professional. Some essential oils may interact with medications, and some people may have an allergic reaction. It's also important to use pure, high-quality essential oils, since some products may have been tampered with or contain chemicals.

Mindful Self-Compassion: How To Cultivate Self-Compassion To Manage Anxiety

Mindful self-compassion is a way of treating yourself with kindness and understanding when things are hard. It is about being mindful of one's own thoughts, feelings, and experiences and treating oneself with the same kindness and understanding that one would offer to a good friend. To use mindful self-compassion to manage anxiety, one can practice mindfulness techniques such as meditation and deep breathing to become more aware of one's thoughts, feelings, and sensations. One can also do self-compassion exercises like writing a letter of kindness to oneself or speaking kindly to oneself when things are hard. Additionally, Self-compassion can also be practiced in daily life by being kind and understanding to oneself and treating oneself with empathy and compassion.

Steps to practicing mindful self-compassion include:

A. **Be present**: Bring your attention to the present moment and acknowledge your feelings, thoughts, and physical sensations without judgment.
B. **Be kind**: Speak to yourself with kindness and understanding, as you would to a friend.
C. **Be aware of common humanity**: Remind yourself that suffering is a universal human experience and that you are not alone in your struggles.
D. **Use self-compassion phrases**: Repeat phrases such as "This is a moment of suffering," "Suffering is a part of life," "May I be kind to myself in this moment," and "May I give myself the compassion that I need."
E. **Practice mindfulness**: Bring a non-judgmental awareness to your feelings and thoughts, recognizing them without getting caught up in them.
F. **Take a compassionate action**: Engage in an act of self-care or self-compassion, such as taking a warm bath or listening to soothing music.
G. **Reflect**: Take a few minutes to reflect on your experience and notice any changes in your anxiety levels or mood.
H. **Repeat**: Incorporate mindful self-compassion into your daily routine and practice it regularly.

Mindful Movement: How To Use Tai Chi And Qigong To Reduce Anxiety

Mindful movement is a form of exercise that combines physical movement with mindfulness practices. Tai chi and Qigong are traditional Chinese practices that involve slow, flowing movements and deep breathing. Both practices have been shown to help reduce anxiety symptoms by making people feel more relaxed, easing muscle tension, and making people feel better overall. To use Tai chi and Qigong to reduce anxiety, one can begin by learning the basic movements and breathing techniques and then incorporating them into a regular practice. It's important to practice often and consistently, ideally for at least 15 to 20 minutes a day. Also, it's best to find a qualified teacher who can help you with your practice and guide you.

How Does Tai Chi Help Reduce Anxiety?

Tai chi is a form of martial arts that is known for its slow, flowing movements, deep breathing, and meditative focus. It is believed to have a positive impact on mental health, including reducing anxiety. The slow, fluid movements and deep breathing can help calm the mind and reduce stress. The meditative focus can also help to increase mindfulness, which can reduce rumination and worry. Some studies have found that practicing tai chi may help reduce symptoms of anxiety and improve overall well-being. The combination of physical movement and meditative focus may also help to make you feel more relaxed and lessen muscle tension, both of which can make anxiety symptoms worse.

Tai Chi is a traditional Chinese martial art that involves slow, fluid movements and deep breathing. Some Tai Chi techniques that may help curb anxiety include:

A. **Slow, flowing movements**: The slow, fluid movements of Tai Chi can help to relax the body and mind, and reduce feelings of tension and stress.

B. **Deep breathing**: Tai Chi incorporates deep breathing techniques, which can help to calm the nervous system and reduce feelings of anxiety.

C. **Focusing on the present moment**: Tai Chi emphasizes being present and mindful in the moment, which can help to reduce worry about the past or future.

D. **Mind-body connection**: Tai chi helps to improve the connection between the mind and body, which can help reduce feelings of anxiety.
E. **Meditative state**: Tai Chi can put the practitioners in a meditative state, which can help to reduce feelings of anxiety by calming the mind and promoting a sense of inner peace.

How Does Qigong Help Reduce Anxiety?

Qigong, like Tai Chi, is a form of mindful movement that combines physical postures, breathing techniques, and meditation. Practicing qigong can help curb anxiety by promoting relaxation, reducing muscle tension, and calming the mind. Qigong can also help regulate the nervous system, which can reduce the physical symptoms of anxiety such as increased heart rate and muscle tension. Additionally, the slow, flowing movements of Qigong can help to focus the mind, which can help to reduce racing thoughts and worry, which are common symptoms of anxiety.

Qigong techniques that may help curb anxiety include:

A. Slow, flowing movements that focus on breathing and relaxation
B. Mindfulness and visualization practices that help to quiet the mind and reduce stress
C. Postures and movements that promote balance and stability in the body
D. Meditative practices that involve concentration and focus on specific points in the body or energy pathways
E. Gentle stretches and massages that help to release tension in the muscles and promote relaxation.

Mindfulness-Based Stress Reduction (MBSR) And Its Effectiveness In Managing Anxiety

Mindfulness-based stress reduction (MBSR) is a mindfulness program that was created by Jon Kabat-Zinn in the 1970s and has been used and studied by many people. Usually, the program is taught as an 8-

week course that combines mindfulness meditation, yoga, and exercises that help you become more aware of your body. The goal of MBSR is to teach individuals how to be present in the moment and respond to stress and difficult situations in a more mindful and intentional way.

MBSR has been found to be effective in managing anxiety as well as a variety of other mental and physical health conditions. Studies have shown that MBSR can lead to big drops in worry, nervousness, and tension, which are all signs of anxiety. The program has also been found to improve mood, reduce stress, and improve overall well-being. Additionally, MBSR has been found to be as effective as cognitive-behavioral therapy (CBT) for reducing anxiety symptoms. Many places offer classes or workshops on MBSR, and you can also learn about it through books, CDs, and online programs.

The techniques used in MBSR include the following:

A. **Mindful breathing**: This involves paying attention to the sensation of breath as it moves in and out of the body. This can help to bring focus to the present moment and reduce racing thoughts.
B. **Body scan**: This involves lying down and bringing awareness to different parts of the body, noticing any sensations or feelings that arise.
C. **Sitting meditation**: This involves sitting in a comfortable position and focusing on the breath or a chosen object, such as a word or phrase.
D. **Yoga**: This involves a series of physical postures, breathing exercises, and meditation, which can help to reduce tension and improve overall well-being.
E. **Informal mindfulness practices**: This includes bringing mindfulness to daily activities such as walking, eating, and doing chores.
F. **Mindful communication**: This involves paying attention to one's own thoughts, feelings and words before speaking.

G. **Loving-kindness meditation**: This is a form of meditation that involves focusing on sending well wishes to oneself and others.

It is important to note that MBSR is not a substitute for traditional medical care or treatment, but rather an adjunct that may be used to help manage symptoms and improve overall well-being.

What Is Acupuncture And How Does It Curb Anxiety

Acupuncture is a form of traditional Chinese medicine in which thin needles are inserted into specific points on the body to stimulate the body's natural healing processes. It is believed to balance the flow of energy, or "qi," throughout the body and promote physical and mental well-being.

Some studies have suggested that acupuncture may be effective in reducing symptoms of anxiety. For example, one study published in the Journal of Anxiety Disorders found that acupuncture was better at reducing the symptoms of generalized anxiety disorder than a control treatment. Researchers have also found that acupuncture may help reduce the symptoms of panic disorder and post-traumatic stress disorder (PTSD). No one knows for sure how acupuncture can help reduce anxiety, but it may have something to do with how neurotransmitters and other chemicals in the brain that control mood are released.

In the case of anxiety, needles are typically placed in acupoints that correspond to the lung, heart, pericardium, and shenmen (spirit gate) meridians. People think that these points help calm and relax the nervous system and keep it in balance. Also, needles can be put in other acupoints that are linked to certain anxiety symptoms, like headaches or heart palpitations.

It is important to remember that acupuncture should only be done by someone who has been trained and given a license. This is to make sure that it is done safely and correctly. It's also important to know that acupuncture is not a replacement for medical treatments that have been proven to work, but it can be a useful addition.

Summary

Mindfulness techniques are different ways to pay attention to the present moment without making judgments about it. These techniques have been found to be effective in managing anxiety symptoms.

One popular mindfulness technique is mindfulness-based stress reduction (MBSR), which is a program that includes practices such as meditation, yoga, and body awareness exercises. MBSR has been found to be effective in reducing symptoms of anxiety and depression.

Other mindfulness techniques that can be used to manage anxiety include:

A. **Diaphragmatic breathing**: This technique involves breathing deeply into the diaphragm, which can help to reduce muscle tension and anxiety.
B. **Progressive muscle relaxation**: This technique involves tensing and then relaxing different muscle groups in the body. It can help to reduce muscle tension and anxiety.
C. **Guided imagery and visualization**: This technique involves creating mental images of peaceful and calming scenes. It can help to reduce anxiety and promote relaxation.
D. **Aromatherapy and essential oils**: Certain essential oils, such as lavender and peppermint, have been found to have a calming effect on the body and can be used to reduce anxiety symptoms.
E. **Mindful self-compassion**: This technique involves treating oneself with kindness and understanding. It can help to promote self-compassion, which can help to reduce anxiety.
F. **Mindful movement**: Tai chi and Qigong are mindful movement practices that involve slow, flowing movements. These practices have been found to be effective in reducing anxiety symptoms.
G. **Acupuncture**: Acupuncture is a traditional Chinese medicine technique that involves the insertion of thin needles into specific

points of the body. It has been found to be effective in reducing anxiety symptoms.

Overall, mindfulness techniques can be a valuable tool for managing anxiety. They can help reduce symptoms of anxiety and promote relaxation. Mindfulness techniques should be used along with other treatments like therapy and medication, and the choice of which to use should depend on the needs and preferences of the person.

APPLYING COGNITIVE BEHAVIORAL THERAPY (CBT) TO CHALLENGE NEGATIVE THOUGHTS AND BELIEFS

What is Cognitive Behavioral Therapy (CBT)?

Cognitive Behavioral Therapy (CBT) is a form of psychotherapy that focuses on the relationship between thoughts, feelings, and behaviors. It is based on the idea that our thoughts and beliefs influence our emotions and actions, and that by changing these thoughts and beliefs, we can change the way we feel and behave.

CBT is a therapy that focuses on reaching a goal. It is usually a short-term treatment that lasts from 8 to 20 sessions. It is a process in which the therapist and client work together. The therapist will help the client find and question negative thoughts and beliefs that are making them anxious.

The therapist will also teach the client different ways to deal with their anxiety, such as relaxation techniques and problem-solving skills.

One of the most important parts of CBT is figuring out and changing what are called "cognitive distortions," which are bad ways of thinking. These include thoughts such as overgeneralization, catastrophizing, and personalization. The therapist will help the client identify these thoughts and provide them with alternative perspectives and coping strategies.

CBT also involves exposure therapy, which is the gradual, systematic exposure to the feared object or situation in order to reduce the anxiety associated with it. This is done in a controlled and safe environment, with the therapist's guidance.

CBT has been studied a lot and is thought to be an effective way to treat panic disorder, social anxiety disorder, and generalized anxiety disorder, among others. It is also used to treat depression and other mental health conditions.

CBT is not just for people who have been diagnosed with an anxiety disorder; it can be helpful for anyone who is experiencing chronic stress or who wants to learn how to manage their thoughts and emotions more effectively.

Understanding The Connection Between Thoughts, Emotions And Behaviors In Anxiety Disorders

In anxiety disorders, there is often a connection between thoughts, emotions, and behaviors. Negative thoughts and beliefs can lead to feelings of anxiety, which in turn can lead to certain behaviors, such as avoidance or self-medication. For example, someone with social anxiety disorder may have a thought such as "I am going to embarrass myself at the party," which may lead to feelings of anxiety and nervousness. This could then lead to avoiding the party altogether.

Cognitive-Behavioral Therapy (CBT) is a therapeutic approach that focuses on identifying and changing these negative thoughts and beliefs in order to reduce the associated anxiety and improve overall functioning. CBT helps individuals identify and challenge unhelpful thoughts, beliefs, and assumptions that contribute to their anxiety and replace them with more balanced and realistic ones. The therapist will teach the individual to observe and identify these thoughts, emotions, and behaviors and to learn how to control and modify them using different strategies.

For example, a person with a phobia may be taught how to gradually expose themselves to the feared object or situation in order to challenge their belief that the situation is dangerous. This can then make people feel less anxious and help them do better in general.

CBT has been studied a lot, and it is thought to be a good way to treat anxiety disorders. It is usually short-term, usually between 8 and 20 sessions, and focuses on teaching individuals the skills they need to manage their anxiety on their own. It can be delivered in individual or group settings and also be done through self-help books and online resources.

How To Identify And Challenge Negative Thoughts And Belief Using CBT Techniques

Most people have negative thought patterns from time to time, but these patterns can become so entrenched that they disrupt relationships, accomplishments, and even well-being.

Cognitive restructuring is a set of therapy techniques that help people see and change harmful ways of thinking.

When destructive and self-defeating thinking patterns emerge, it's a good idea to look into strategies to interrupt and redirect them. That is what cognitive reorganization is capable of.

What Is The Process Of Cognitive Restructuring?

Cognitive restructuring is at the heart of cognitive behavioral therapy, a well-studied form of talk therapy that has been shown to help with a wide range of mental health problems, such as depression and anxiety disorders.

A patient and therapist collaborate in cognitive behavioral therapy (CBT) to uncover erroneous thought patterns that are contributing to a problem and practice procedures to help alter unfavorable thought patterns.

Recognizing flaws in your own cognitive processes might be difficult. As a result, most professionals advise working with a therapist while beginning cognitive restructuring.

Cognitive restructuring approaches, as the name implies, deconstruct problematic concepts and rebuild them in a more balanced and correct manner.

Cognitive distortions are ways of thinking that cause some people to have a distorted and harmful view of reality. Cognitive distortions are frequently associated with melancholy, anxiety, relational issues, and self-defeating behaviors.

Cognitive distortions include the following:

- Black-and-white thinking.
- Catastrophizing.
- Overgeneralizing.
- Personalizing.

Cognitive restructuring allows you to catch these maladaptive beliefs as they happen. Then you can try reframing these views in more truthful and beneficial ways.

The argument goes that if you can modify your perspective on specific events or circumstances, you may be able to change your sentiments and actions.

So, how can one reconstruct a negative thought?

Techniques For Cognitive Reorganization

Anyone can use cognitive restructuring techniques to change the way they think, but many people find it helpful to work with a therapist.

A therapist can assist you in identifying which cognitive distortions are harming you. They can also explain why or how a thought is unreasonable or incorrect.

A therapist can also teach you how to "challenge" negative thought patterns and redesign them to be more positive.

Here's a quick rundown of some of the cognitive restructuring strategies:

1. Self-Monitoring

To modify an unproductive mental pattern, you must first recognize the error you're making. For cognitive reorganization to work, you have to be able to recognize the thoughts that lead to bad feelings and states of mind.

It's also helpful to keep track of when and where the thoughts arise. You may be more susceptible to cognitive distortions in certain conditions. Knowing what those situations are will help you plan ahead of time.

For example, if you have anxiety and are a student, you might tend to catastrophize when you have an exam. Perhaps your pattern looks like this: "I am certain that I will fail this test, fail the course, and be unable to graduate with the rest of the class." Everyone will realize I've failed.

Knowing that you are weak can help you notice a bad thought and change it before it gets out of hand.

Some people find that journaling as part of the process is beneficial. Even if you're not sure what's causing your worry or unhappiness at first, writing down your thoughts may help you identify a cognitive distortion or pattern.

As you practice self-monitoring, you'll likely become more aware of skewed thought patterns.

2. Questioning Your Assumptions

Another important part of cognitive restructuring is learning to look at your beliefs and assumptions, especially those that seem to get in the way of you living a productive life.

A therapist can teach you how to use the Socratic method of questioning to determine where and how your automatic ideas are biased or unreasonable.

You could ask yourself the following questions:

A. Is this an emotional or factual thought?
B. What proof do you have that this concept is correct?
C. What proof do you have that this concept is incorrect?
D. How could I put my conviction to the test?
E. What could possibly go wrong? How would I react if the worst were to happen?
F. What alternative interpretations could this information have?
G. Is this a black-and-white scenario, or are there shades of grey?

Catastrophizing is a way of thinking that can make you think that the worst possible thing will happen in a stressful situation. You could test this cognitive pattern by listing every possible outcome. You could consider the likelihood of each probable scenario.

When you ask questions, you can think about other possibilities that aren't as bad as the ones you might be afraid of.

3. Gathering Evidence

Gathering evidence is an important part of cognitive reorganization.

You may want to keep track of the circumstances that cause a reaction, such as who you were with and what you were doing. You might want to keep track of how powerful each response is and what memories arise as a result.

You may also gather evidence to support or refute your opinions, assumptions, and beliefs. Cognitive distortions are erroneous and biased, but they can also be profoundly ingrained. Dislodging and replacing them necessitates evidence of their rationality.

You might need to make a list of facts that show a belief is true and compare it to facts that show the belief is wrong or just not true.

For example, if you personalize the behavior of others, you may frequently blame yourself for things that are not your fault. It might help to look at data that shows an action has nothing to do with you.

4. Performing A Cost-Benefit Analysis

Using this method, you would figure out if keeping a certain cognitive distortion is worth it or not by weighing its pros and cons.

You could think to yourself:

A. What good does it do to proclaim yourself a complete moron, for example?
B. How much does this thought pattern cost you emotionally and practically?
C. What are the long-term consequences?

D. What effect does this thought pattern have on those around you?

E. How does it help or hinder your job performance?

Putting the pros and cons next to each other can help you decide if it's worth it to change the pattern.

Here's an example of a recent celebrity using a cost-benefit analysis:

Hannah Gadsby, a comedian, spoke on her program "Nanette" about how she built a career on self-deprecating humor. But, at some point, the damage she was doing to her self-esteem exceeded the benefits of her job. So she resolved to quit tearing herself down to make jokes.

"Nanette" was a huge success, thanks in part to the fact that so many people understand the terrible trade-offs they make every day.

5. Generating Alternatives

Cognitive restructuring helps people find new ways to look at the things that happen to them. Part of the technique is coming up with logical and helpful explanations to replace the misunderstandings that have grown over time.

For example, if you didn't perform well on a test, instead of concluding that you're bad at arithmetic, you should look at ways to improve your study habits. You might also look into some relaxing techniques to attempt before your next test.

Another example: If a group of colleagues stops talking when you walk into the room, rather than assuming they are talking about you, you might want to consider other possibilities. You may learn that the incident had nothing to do with you or that you misread what was going on as a result of doing so.

Another way to come up with alternatives is to replace wrong or unhelpful thought patterns with positive affirmations.

You should remind yourself that you make valuable, positive contributions at work and that your coworkers always include you in what's going on. You can base these on a list of real things you've done to help others and good relationships you've made.

What are the Benefits?

Although working with a therapist is beneficial at first, cognitive restructuring is a practice that you can learn to do on your own once you understand how it works.

There are numerous advantages to being able to recognize and change negative thought patterns. For example, it may be beneficial to:

- Reduce your stress and anxiety.
- Improve your communication skills and cultivate healthier relationships
- Substitute unhealthy coping mechanisms such as substance abuse
- Rebuild self-esteem and confidence

What Problems Might Cognitive Restructuring Help With?

CBT is recommended by the American Psychological Association to help with:

- Eating problems
- Melancholy
- Stress
- PTSD
- Substance abuse problem
- Mental illness
- Marriage issues

It can also assist you through tough transitions such as divorce, a significant illness, or the death of a loved one.

Cognitive restructuring can help you challenge and change unhelpful thoughts in any situation where you tend to think negatively.

Are there any drawbacks?

Because it is recommended that clients work with a therapist, one possible disadvantage of cognitive restructuring could be the out-of-pocket financial cost of treatment sessions.

Mayo Clinic doctors believe that in some circumstances, CBT procedures are most helpful when paired with medication.

The Bottom Line

One of the cornerstones of cognitive behavioral therapy is cognitive restructuring.

Cognitive reorganization is usually collaborative. A therapist and a patient often work together to find and change unhealthy thought patterns with healthier, more honest ways of looking at events and situations.

Cognitive restructuring can help with anxiety and depression symptoms, as well as a variety of other mental health disorders.

The Role Of Journaling And Thought Records In CBT

Cognitive behavioral therapy (CBT) uses journaling and keeping track of thoughts as important tools to help people find and change their negative thoughts and beliefs. Journaling is the process of writing down one's thoughts, feelings, and experiences. It can be used to monitor mood and behavior patterns as well as for self-reflection.

Thought records, also known as thought journals, are a specific type of journaling used in CBT. They involve writing down a hard situation, the negative thoughts and beliefs that came up in response to it, and the evidence for and against those thoughts. This process helps people see and question their negative thoughts and beliefs, so they can think in a more balanced and realistic way.

Both journaling and thought records are used as part of CBT to help individuals recognize patterns in their thoughts and behaviors and to develop new ways of thinking about and reacting to situations. People with different kinds of anxiety disorders, such as panic disorder, phobias, social anxiety disorder, and generalized anxiety disorder, can use these techniques to get better.

Behavioral Techniques: How To Change Actions And Behaviors That Reinforce Negative Thoughts And Beliefs

In cognitive-behavioral therapy (CBT), one of the behavioral techniques is to change actions and behaviors that make negative thoughts and beliefs stronger. The goal of these techniques is to find unhealthy patterns of behavior and replace them with healthier, more adaptive ones. Examples of behavioral techniques include:

A. **Exposure therapy**: Gradually exposing the person to feared situations or stimuli in a controlled setting with the goal of reducing fear and anxiety over time.

B. **Activity scheduling**: Planning and engaging in specific activities or tasks to increase positive experiences and decrease avoidance behaviors.

C. **Relaxation techniques**: Teaching the person coping strategies to manage physical symptoms of anxiety such as deep breathing, progressive muscle relaxation, and visualization.

D. **Social skills training**: Teaching the person how to interact with others in a more effective way to improve social functioning and reduce social anxiety

E. **Problem-solving**: Teaching the person how to identify, analyze, and solve problems in a more effective way to reduce stress and anxiety

These techniques are often used with cognitive techniques, like noticing and questioning negative thoughts and beliefs, to help change the thought processes that lead to anxiety disorders.

Mindfulness And CBT: How To Incorporate Mindfulness Into CBT To Challenge Negative Thoughts And Beliefs

CBT and mindfulness are both good ways to deal with anxiety disorders, and they can be used together to challenge negative thoughts and beliefs. Mindfulness is the practice of being present and aware in the moment, without judgment. It involves paying attention to one's thoughts, emotions, and physical sensations without getting caught up in them. On the other hand, CBT is a form of therapy that focuses on identifying and changing negative thoughts and beliefs that contribute to anxiety.

To add mindfulness to CBT, a therapist might lead a client through mindfulness exercises like deep breathing and body scanning, which help people become more aware of their thoughts and feelings. This awareness can then be used to challenge negative thoughts and beliefs. For example, if a client is anxious because they think they are not good enough, they might be taught to watch this thought without judging it and to question whether or not it is true. They might be told to look at things from different points of view and pay attention to the present.

Behavior techniques like exposure therapy, which involves gradually exposing a person to the thing they are afraid of and making them less afraid of it, can also be used to change actions and behaviors that reinforce negative thoughts and beliefs.

Journaling and thought records are also often used in CBT as a way to track and identify negative thoughts, beliefs, and patterns. This allows clients to become more aware of these thoughts and beliefs and to challenge them more effectively.

Overall, adding mindfulness to CBT can help clients become more aware of their thoughts and feelings, challenge negative beliefs, and change behaviors that reinforce these beliefs. This can lead to a decrease in anxiety symptoms.

The Role Of Homework And Daily Practice In CBT

In cognitive behavioral therapy (CBT), doing homework and practicing every day are important parts of getting better. Therapists often give clients homework to help them put what they've learned in therapy to use in their daily lives. Clients can keep working on their goals and improving their mental health outside of therapy by practicing every day.

Examples of homework assignments in CBT can include:

- Keeping a thought diary to identify and challenge negative thoughts
- Practicing relaxation techniques such as deep breathing or progressive muscle relaxation
- Completing exposure therapy exercises to confront feared situations or objects
- Practicing cognitive restructuring techniques to challenge negative beliefs and replace them with more positive and realistic ones

By completing their homework and engaging in daily practice, clients can develop the skills and strategies necessary to manage their anxiety disorder effectively. This can lead to an increase in self-awareness and self-confidence, as well as help clients see progress in therapy, which can be a powerful motivator to continue working on their goals.

Using Visualization and Imagery in CBT to Challenge Negative Thoughts and Beliefs

Cognitive Behavioral Therapy (CBT) is a form of psychotherapy that aims to change negative thoughts, emotions, and behaviors that may be contributing to an individual's anxiety disorder. One way to do this is through the use of visualization and imagery.

This method involves imagining a good outcome or what you want to happen and then using that image to challenge negative thoughts and beliefs. For example, if someone is afraid of public speaking, they might use visualization and imagery to imagine giving a presentation in front of a large group of people and making it go well. By imagining this, the person can challenge their negative thoughts about their ability to speak in public and start to develop a more positive and realistic outlook. Visualization and imagery can also be used to practice ways to deal with anxiety, such as deep breathing or progressive muscle relaxation. It's important to note that visualization and imagery should be done with the guidance of a therapist or counselor who is trained in CBT techniques.

Conclusion

Cognitive-Behavioral Therapy (CBT) is a form of psychotherapy that focuses on the connection between thoughts, emotions, and behaviors. The key principle of CBT is that negative thoughts and beliefs can lead to negative emotions and behaviors, which can then reinforce those negative thoughts and beliefs. To break this cycle, CBT techniques are used to identify and challenge negative thoughts and beliefs and change the actions and behaviors that reinforce them.

One way to use mindfulness in CBT is to pay attention to the present and watch thoughts and feelings without judging them. This can help to decrease the power that negative thoughts and beliefs have over a person.

One CBT technique to challenge negative thoughts and beliefs is the use of journaling and thought records. This means writing down negative thoughts and beliefs as they come up and then looking for evidence for and against them to challenge them. This can help identify patterns and correct any inaccuracies in thinking.

You can also change actions and behaviors that support negative thoughts and beliefs by using techniques like exposure therapy and relaxation. Exposure therapy, for example, gradually puts a person in a situation they are afraid of. Deep breathing and relaxing your muscles one at a time are two ways to relax that can help lessen the physical effects of anxiety.

Homework and daily practice are essential parts of CBT. This means doing things like keeping a journal or record of your thoughts, going through exposure therapy, and learning how to relax. The goal is to make the techniques a part of daily life so that they can be used in real-life situations to deal with negative thoughts and beliefs.

Using visualization and imagery in CBT involves creating a mental image of a positive outcome and using this image to challenge negative thoughts and beliefs. For example, if a person has a negative belief about their ability to speak in public, they can visualize themselves giving a successful presentation. This can help to replace negative thoughts and beliefs with positive ones.

In summary, CBT is a form of psychotherapy that focuses on the connection between thoughts, emotions, and behaviors. By using techniques such as journaling and thought records, exposure therapy, relaxation techniques, visualization and imagery, and daily practice, CBT can help to change negative thoughts, beliefs, actions, and behaviors that reinforce them. Incorporating mindfulness into CBT can help to decrease the power that negative thoughts and beliefs have over a person and help them develop a more balanced perspective on their thoughts and emotions.

THE IMPORTANCE OF EXERCISE AND NUTRITION IN MANAGING ANXIETY

Exercise and nutrition play an important role in managing anxiety. Regular exercise and a healthy diet can help reduce the physical symptoms of anxiety, like tense muscles and a fast heartbeat, and can also improve your overall mood and mental health.

Exercise has been shown to be an effective treatment for anxiety. It releases endorphins, which are chemicals in the brain that act as natural painkillers and mood elevators. Exercise also helps new brain cells grow and makes the brain better at processing information. Regular exercise has also been shown to make it less likely that someone will get an anxiety disorder or feel down.

Nutrition is also important for managing anxiety. A healthy diet with a variety of fruits, vegetables, whole grains, lean proteins, and healthy fats can give the body the nutrients it needs to work well. A diet high in sugar and caffeine can increase anxiety symptoms. Eating a well-balanced diet can help you feel better, have more energy, and feel less anxious.

Getting regular exercise and eating well can help you deal with anxiety in a natural and effective way. Before starting an exercise or nutrition plan, it's important to talk to a doctor or nurse, especially if the person already has health problems.

Additionally, it is important to note that the relationship between nutrition and anxiety is complex, and more research is needed to fully understand the mechanisms at play. But it's clear that a healthy diet and regular physical activity can help reduce anxiety symptoms and make you feel better overall.

Understanding the Link Between Physical Activity, Nutrition, and Anxiety

There is a strong link between physical activity, nutrition, and anxiety. Regular exercise has been shown to reduce anxiety symptoms and improve mental health in general. Exercise can help to release endorphins, which are chemicals in the brain that promote feelings of well-being and reduce stress. Exercise can also help with sleep, which is often disturbed in anxious people.

Proper nutrition is also important for managing anxiety. Eating a well-balanced diet that includes plenty of fruits, vegetables, whole grains, and lean protein can help provide the body with the nutrients it needs to function properly. Additionally, avoiding processed foods, caffeine, and alcohol can also help reduce anxiety symptoms.

Certain vitamins and minerals, such as omega-3 fatty acids, vitamin D, and magnesium, have been linked to reducing symptoms of anxiety.

In conclusion, a healthy diet and regular physical activity can work together to improve mental health and lessen anxiety symptoms. Engaging in regular exercise and making healthy food choices can provide the body with the nutrients it needs to function properly while reducing stress and promoting feelings of well-being.

The Benefits Of Regular Exercise For Managing Anxiety

Exercise is typically the last thing on your mind when you are depressed or anxious. However, once motivated, exercise can have a significant effect.

Exercise can help prevent and treat a variety of health issues, including high blood pressure, diabetes, and arthritis. According to studies on depression, anxiety, and exercise, the psychological and physical advantages of exercise can help improve mood and reduce worry.

Even though there aren't clear links between depression, anxiety, and exercise, it's clear that working out and other forms of physical activity can help you feel better and lessen the effects of depression or anxiety. Exercise may also help keep depression and anxiety at bay once you've recovered.

How Does Exercise Aid In The Treatment Of Depression And Anxiety?

Regular exercise can help with depression and anxiety by doing the following:

- Enhancing your sensation of well-being by releasing feel-good endorphins, natural cannabis-like brain chemicals (endogenous cannabinoids), and other natural brain chemicals.
- Distracting yourself from anxieties in order to break the loop of negative thoughts that feed sadness and anxiety.

Regular exercise also provides numerous psychological and emotional benefits. It can assist you in the following ways:

1. **Develop self-assurance**. Meeting workout objectives or challenges, no matter how minor, can increase your self-esteem. Getting in shape might also help you feel better about yourself.

2. **Increase your social engagement**. Exercise and physical exercise may provide you with the opportunity to meet and socialize with others. Simply exchanging a polite grin or hello, while walking around your neighborhood, can improve your attitude.

3. **Deal with stress in a healthy way**. A healthy coping method is to do something positive to deal with depression or anxiety. Drinking alcohol to feel better, concentrating on how you feel, or thinking sadness or anxiety would go away on its own can all lead to increased symptoms.

Is scheduled exercise your only option?

According to some studies, regular physical activity, such as walking, rather than just structured training regimens, may improve mood. Physical activity and exercise are not synonymous, although both are good for your health.

Physical exercise is any activity that uses your muscles and uses up energy. This could be something you do at work, at home, or for fun.

Exercise is any activity that the body does over and over again that is planned, structured, and done in a certain way to get or stay fit.

The word "exercise" may conjure up images of running laps around the gym. But exercise is a broad term for a lot of different things that make you more active and feel better.

Running, lifting weights, playing basketball, and other heart-pumping physical activities can all assist. Some less strenuous activities that can help are gardening, washing your car, walking around the block, and so on. Any physical exercise that gets you up and moving will help you feel better.

You do not have to complete all of your exercise or physical activity at once. Change the way you think about exercise and look for ways to do small amounts of physical activity all day long. Take the stairs instead of the elevator, for example. To fit in a quick stroll, park a bit further away from work. Consider riding to work if you live close to your workplace.

How Much Of Physical Activity Is Enough?

Exercise for 30 minutes or more, three to five days a week, may significantly reduce depression or anxiety symptoms. Smaller quantities of physical activity, such as 10 to 15 minutes at a time, may have an impact. Exercise that is more vigorous, such as jogging or bicycling, may take less time to boost your mood.

The mental health benefits of exercise and physical activity may only continue if you stay with them over time, which is another reason to prioritize choosing things that you enjoy.

How do I get started—and stay motivated?

Starting and maintaining an exercise plan or regular physical activity can be difficult. These steps may be useful:

1. Determine what you enjoy doing. Determine the types of physical activities you're most likely to engage in, and consider when and how you're most likely to follow through. On example, would you rather garden in the evening, start your day with a jog, go for a bike trip, or play hoops with your children after school? Do something you enjoy to keep you motivated.

2. Seek the advice of a mental health professional. Seek advice and assistance from your doctor or a mental health professional. Discuss a physical activity or exercise regimen and how it fits into your overall treatment plan.

3. Establish attainable objectives. Your goal does not have to be to walk for an hour five days a week. Consider what you might be able to do realistically and start slowly. Rather than setting unrealistic limits that you are unlikely to reach, tailor your plan to your individual requirements and talents.

Don't consider exercise or physical activity to be a duty. You'll link exercise with failure if it's just another "should" in your life that you don't believe you're meeting. Rather, think of your exercise or physical activity program in the same way that you think of your therapy sessions or medication—as one of the instruments that will help you get better.

4. Examine your roadblocks. Determine what is preventing you from being physically active or exercising. If you are self-conscious, you might wish to exercise at home. Find a friend to work out with or who appreciates the same physical activities that you do if you stick to objectives better with a partner. If you don't have money to spend on fitness equipment, try something free, like daily walking. If you consider what is preventing you from being physically active or exercising, you will most likely find an alternative answer.

5. Be prepared for setbacks and roadblocks. Give yourself credit for every modest move in the right direction. If you skip a day of exercise, it doesn't mean you can't maintain an exercise routine and should give up. Simply try again the following day. Continue to do so.

Is It Necessary That I See A Doctor?

Talk to your doctor before you start a new exercise plan to make sure it's safe for you. Talk to your doctor to find out what activities, how much exercise, and what intensity level are right for you. Your doctor will take into account whatever medications you are taking as well as your medical history. He or she may also have suggestions for getting started and remaining motivated.

If you work out regularly but still feel depressed or anxious, talk to your doctor or a mental health professional. Exercise and physical activity are excellent strategies to alleviate depression and anxiety symptoms, but they are not a substitute for talk therapy (psychotherapy) or pharmaceuticals.

How To Create An Effective Exercise Plan For Managing Anxiety

Creating an effective exercise plan for managing anxiety involves several key steps. First, it's important to set specific, measurable, and realistic goals for your exercise routine. This could be something as simple as committing to 30 minutes of physical activity each day or increasing your overall fitness level.

Next, it's important to choose activities that you enjoy and that align with your fitness level. This can include anything from going for a walk or jog to swimming, cycling, or participating in a fitness class.

It's also important to consider the timing of your exercise routine. Research suggests that getting some exercise in the morning or early afternoon may help with anxiety symptoms the most.

Also, it's important to talk to a doctor or nurse before starting an exercise plan, especially if you already have health problems. They can help you create a safe and effective plan that's tailored to your needs.

Regular exercise is important for dealing with anxiety because it releases endorphins, which are natural mood boosters, and lowers stress and tension in the body. Regular physical activity can also help you sleep better, which can help you deal with anxiety symptoms.

The Role Of Cardio And Strength Training In Managing Anxiety

Cardio- or aerobic-type exercise, such as running, cycling, or swimming, increases the heart rate and blood flow, releasing endorphins, also known as "feel-good" hormones. This can help improve your mood and reduce feelings of anxiety. Also, cardio exercise can help you sleep better and feel less stressed, both of which can make you anxious.

Strength training, like lifting weights or doing exercises with your own body, has also been shown to help with anxiety. Neurotransmitters like serotonin and dopamine are made more of when you do this kind of exercise. This can improve your mood and make you feel less anxious. Strength training can also help improve self-esteem and body image, two things that can be hurt by anxiety.

Creating an effective exercise plan for managing anxiety starts with setting realistic goals and finding activities that are enjoyable and sustainable. Five times a week, you should try to get at least 30 minutes of moderate-intensity exercise, like brisk walking. But it's important to talk to a doctor or nurse before starting a new exercise plan, especially if you already have health problems.

Top Seven Exercises for Anxiety Disorders

Anxiety and depression are the two most common mental illnesses in the United States. These medical disorders currently affect more than 40 million adults in the United States.

Regardless of how common these conditions are, exercise can help you cope with them and lessen their negative influence on your life.

We've produced a list of the top seven workouts for anxiety and sadness!

1. Jogging

Running is an excellent way to clear your mind and relieve tension. These two characteristics can aid in the reduction of anxiety and despair.

While over 550,000 individuals participate in marathons each year, you don't have to run that far to reap the benefits of this type of training. Running is a terrific way to get away from your everyday routine and focus on yourself.

Life's day-to-day concerns can sometimes cause additional stress. These factors can increase anxiety and lead to depression. Running for at least 30 minutes forces you to do anything other than focus on what's bothering you.

2. Yoga

Yoga is a popular type of exercise that combines physical activity with regulated breathing.

Meditation and core movements are both parts of a yoga routine that can help you feel better emotionally and physically. Another thing that makes yoga unique is that you can do it by yourself or with a group.

Yoga with others might help you stay on track with your workout routine. It can also surround you with other like-minded people who may be experiencing some of the same anxiety and depression symptoms that you are.

This can help you build a useful network of support to help you get through good and bad days.

3. Trekking

Hiking in the woods is a terrific way to get away from it all while connecting with nature.

Being in the woods removes you from the hustle and bustle of everyday life and places you in a tranquil and serene atmosphere. Hiking might be difficult depending on where you live due to height gain and other weather factors.

The peace and quiet of the woods can make it the perfect place to relax and enjoy nature while getting some exercise. Hiking, like other forms of exercise, boosts blood flow to your brain and muscles, which might release endorphins that make you feel good!

4. Bodybuilding

Weightlifting is a great way to keep your body in good shape and improve your mental health.

Depression can sometimes be brought on by a painful event in your life or by gaining weight that you don't want to have. Lifting weights will provide you with a physical challenge while also assisting you in releasing rage or other forms of aggression that are hidden beneath the surface.

This is especially beneficial after a long and stressful day at home or at work.

5. Go for long walks

A long stroll can help you clear your mind while also enhancing your physical health.

Walking 10,000 steps per day equals around five miles and is an excellent daily goal to establish for yourself. People may sometimes make excuses for not meeting their daily walking goals. These frequently involve being "overburdened" with work, education, or family.

Don't jeopardize your mental health by making excuses for yourself. Dedicate yourself to taking long walks so that you can meet your daily step goal. While 10,000 is an excellent goal to strive for, you may need to begin your walks with a lower goal in mind.

While taking these walks, encourage yourself to think about topics other than what is giving you anxiety or depression. It can be a saving grace to use this time to focus on other things!

6. Swimming

Swimming is one of the best kinds of exercise and can be one of your most effective weapons in combating depression and anxiety symptoms. It's also an excellent exercise to do in the summer if you live in a hot region where the heat can be dangerous.

Swimming forces you to take deeper breaths and works out both small and large muscles that you might not use often outside of the water. It's also a sort of workout that will help you keep your flexibility without harming your bones and joints.

Unlike running, which can strain your knees and ankles due to the hard surface, swimming in a pool produces resistance while also moving with your muscles.

Pool workouts can help you overcome anxiety and sadness while also improving your aerobic health!

7. Dancing

Dancing may not be the first exercise that comes to mind when considering strategies to combat melancholy and anxiety, but its health advantages cannot be overlooked.

There are numerous types of dancing, and some of the faster-paced dances can provide an excellent physical workout. Dancing is not only an aerobic activity, but it is also a lot of fun. You can do it with a partner or in a group while listening to your favorite songs.

You can also set a goal for yourself to learn new dance genres and reward yourself for mastering new moves. These incentives can help you obtain the confidence you need to overcome the severe symptoms of anxiety and depression.

Anxiety and depression can induce mental and physical symptoms that impair your regular activities. You may notice that you are no longer enjoying routine activities or that you feel distant from the people around you.

It's crucial to realize that millions of individuals throughout the world are suffering from the same problem. Exercise is one approach to boost your mental health while also keeping your physical state and well-being in check.

The Impact Of Diet And Nutrition On Anxiety

Diet and nutrition play a significant role in managing anxiety. Consuming a balanced diet that includes a variety of fruits, vegetables, lean proteins, and whole grains can help to reduce symptoms of anxiety. These types of foods provide the necessary nutrients for the body to function properly, including vitamins, minerals, and antioxidants, which can help to lower inflammation and improve overall health.

On the other hand, consuming a diet high in processed foods, sugar, and caffeine can increase symptoms of anxiety. These types of foods can cause blood sugar fluctuations, which can lead to feelings of irritability, restlessness, and nervousness. Additionally, caffeine can cause increased heart rate and jitteriness, which can worsen anxiety symptoms.

Certain nutrients have been found to be particularly beneficial for managing anxiety. These include omega-3 fatty acids, magnesium, and B vitamins. Omega-3 fatty acids, found in fatty fish such as salmon and tuna, as well as in flaxseeds, chia seeds and walnuts, have been shown to decrease inflammation and improve brain function, which can help to reduce symptoms of anxiety. Magnesium, found in leafy greens, nuts, and seeds, can help to relax the muscles and calm the mind, which can also reduce anxiety symptoms. B vitamins, found in fruits, vegetables, and whole grains, are important for maintaining healthy brain function and can also help to reduce anxiety symptoms.

In summary, eating a balanced diet that includes a variety of nutrient-rich foods while avoiding processed foods, sugar, and caffeine can help to reduce symptoms of anxiety. Additionally, including foods that are rich in omega-3 fatty acids, magnesium, and B vitamins can help provide additional support for managing anxiety.

The Importance Of A Balanced Diet In Managing Anxiety

The National Institute of Mental Health says that anxiety disorders are the most common type of mental illness in the United States. Anxiety affects 40 million adults, or 18% of the population. Depression and anxiety are often found together, and about half of people with depression also have anxiety.

Anxiety can be made easier to deal with with certain therapies and drugs, but only about one-third of people who have it go to therapy. But when talking about the different ways to treat anxiety, nutrition is a very important part of the picture.

A diet high in whole grains, vegetables, and fruits is a better choice than a diet high in simple carbs found in processed foods. It is also vital to consider when you eat. You should not miss meals. This could cause your blood sugar to drop, which can make you feel nervous and make your anxiety worse if you already have it.

The gut-brain axis is also particularly important because the gut lining contains a large percentage (approximately 95%) of serotonin receptors. Probiotics are being studied for their potential to relieve anxiety and depression.

Diets That Can Assist You Curb Anxiety

It may surprise you to find that certain foods have been proven to reduce anxiety.

A. In mice, diets lacking in magnesium were found to promote anxiety-related behaviors. Natural magnesium-rich foods may help a person feel calmer. Examples include leafy greens such as spinach and Swiss chard. Moreover, legumes, nuts, seeds, and whole grains are also good sources.

B. Zinc-rich foods like oysters, cashews, liver, beef, and egg yolks have been related to reduced anxiety.

C. Other foods that contain omega-3 fatty acids include fatty seafood such as wild Alaskan salmon. One of the earliest studies, conducted on medical students in 2011, found that omega-3 fatty acids may help lower anxiety. (Omega-3 fatty acid supplements were employed in this study). Prior to the study, omega-3 fatty acids had only been associated to depression relief.

D. A study published in the journal Psychiatry Research found a relationship between probiotic diets and reduced social anxiety. Probiotic-rich foods like pickles, sauerkraut, and kefir have been associated to reduced symptoms.

E. Asparagus is a well-known nutritious veggie. Because of its anti-anxiety effects, the Chinese government allowed the use of asparagus extract as a natural functional food and beverage component based on studies.

F. Avocados and almonds, because they are high in B vitamins.

G. These "feel-good" foods stimulate the release of neurotransmitters like serotonin and dopamine. They are a simple and safe initial step in dealing with anxiety.

Should You Incorporate Antioxidants In Your Anti-Anxiety Diet

Anxiety is known to be associated with a decrease in total antioxidant status. It stands to reason, then, that increasing your intake of antioxidant-rich foods may help alleviate the symptoms of anxiety disorders. In 2010, a study looked at the antioxidant levels of 3,100 foods, spices, plants, drinks, and supplements. The USDA lists the following foods as high in antioxidants:

- Dried little red, pinto, black, and red kidney beans.
- Fruits such as Gala, Granny Smith, and Red Delicious apples, prunes, sweet cherries, plums, and black plums

- Berries such as Blackberries, strawberries, cranberries, raspberries, and blueberries.
- Nuts such as walnuts and pecans.
- Vegetable such as Artichokes, kale, spinach, beets, and broccoli.
- Spices such as turmeric (which contains the active chemical curcumin) and ginger. These two spices have both antioxidant and anti-anxiety qualities.

Improving Mental Wellness Through Eating

Talk to your doctor if your anxiety symptoms are severe or if they last for more than two weeks. Even if your doctor advises medicine or counseling for anxiety, it is worth considering whether you might also benefit from dietary changes. While nutritional psychiatry is not a replacement for other treatments, the connection between diet, mood, and anxiety is receiving more attention. There is a growing body of evidence, but more research is needed to properly grasp the significance of nutritional psychiatry, or psycho-nutrition, as I prefer to call it.

There are numerous other dietary factors that can help relieve anxiety, in addition to healthy standards such as eating a balanced diet, drinking enough water to stay hydrated, and limiting or eliminating alcohol and caffeine. Complex carbs, for example, are broken down more slowly and help keep your blood sugar level more stable, which makes you feel better.

The Role Of Omega-3 Fatty Acids, Vitamins And Minerals In Managing Anxiety

Omega-3 fatty acids, vitamins, and minerals have been shown to have a positive impact on managing anxiety. Omega-3 fatty acids, specifically EPA and DHA, are found in fish such as salmon, mackerel, and sardines and in supplements such as fish oil. They have been found to have anti-inflammatory effects and may help reduce symptoms of anxiety and depression.

Some vitamins, like the B vitamins, especially vitamin B12 and folate, have also been shown to help with anxiety. Vitamin B12 helps with the production of neurotransmitters, which are chemicals in the brain that regulate mood. Folate, also known as vitamin B9, is important for the production of neurotransmitters and has been shown to be effective in reducing symptoms of anxiety and depression.

Minerals such as magnesium and zinc have also been found to be important for managing anxiety. Magnesium is important because it helps control neurotransmitters, especially GABA, which is known to calm the brain. Zinc is important for the production of neurotransmitters and has been found to be low in people with anxiety disorders.

In addition to the above, a balanced diet with the right amount of fruits and vegetables, lean protein, healthy fats, and whole grains is important for managing anxiety. Avoiding processed foods and foods high in sugar and caffeine is also important. Drinking water and staying hydrated are also important for managing anxiety.

It is important to note that everyone's nutritional needs are different, and it is recommended to consult a healthcare professional or a registered dietitian to create a personalized diet plan that will best fit your needs.

Understanding Omega-3 In Your Quest To Curbing Anxiety Disorders

We adjust our diets throughout our lives to meet the demands of our unique lifestyles, with dramatic shifts from childhood to adulthood. Without a doubt, this is necessary for growth, physical functioning, and cognitive activity. While our diet evolves to support these processes, some staple nutrients should remain stable throughout time. Some vitamins and minerals that come to mind are vitamin C, vitamin B12, or even calcium; nevertheless, the lesser-known omega-3 fatty acid is an important contributor to human health.

Omega-3 is well known for its ability to reduce inflammation, but it also helps us fight disease and improve our overall health in a number of other ways. Omega-3 has a wide range of functions, from preventing and treating heart disease to preserving our eyesight from degenerative disorders. Perhaps the most impressive function is its impact on numerous mental health issues, particularly anxiety disorders. Omega-3, a vital component found in a variety of foods, could be a simple yet healthful supplement to typical prescription-based approaches to treating anxiety problems.

Before we go any further, let's get acquainted with this fatty acid.

Omega-3 Fatty Acids: An Overview

Omega-3 is a polyunsaturated fatty acid, which means it has numerous double bonds in its structure and is therefore a good type of fat. It can be either a short-chain fatty acid with 18 or fewer carbon atoms or a long-chain fatty acid with at least 20 or more carbon atoms, depending on the kind of omega-3 fat.

Omega-3 fatty acids contribute to human health and lifespan by fighting disease, preventing malfunctions, and promoting good health on a systemic level. It accomplishes this in a variety of ways, including:

- Reducing risk factors for heart disease by lowering blood pressure, lowering the incidence of blood clots, increasing HDL ("good" cholesterol), and so on.
- Fighting local and systemic inflammation, which aids in the treatment of a variety of autoimmune disorders (such as rheumatoid arthritis and lupus)
- Promoting brain health during pregnancy and early childhood.
- Protecting against age-related mental deterioration, such as Alzheimer's disease.
- Preventing mental illnesses such as anxiety and sadness.

Omega-3 Food Sources

Unfortunately, our bodies can't make omega-3 on their own, even though it is an important part of a healthy diet. We must instead complement this source through nutrition. Fish and fish oils (particularly fatty fish like salmon or sardines), as well as nuts and seeds, are good sources of omega-3 lipids (such as flaxseed, chia seeds, and walnuts).

Supplementing with tablets or pills may be a good option for those who are less willing to replace their omega-3 levels through these food sources. Consult your doctor to identify the best course of action for you.

The Different Types of Omega-3 Fatty Acids

A. Alpha-linoleic Acid (ALA).

The most frequent omega-3 fatty acid in our diet is ALA. It is found in foods such as flax seeds, flaxseed oil, chia seeds, walnuts, and other nuts and seeds. Our bodies turn ALA straight into energy, and it can only serve this purpose until it is converted into one of the two other forms of omega-3 fats (EPA or DHA). This translation takes place by means of biological processes involving various beginning molecules, enzymes, and cofactors. This translation is impossible without all of the nutrients and enzymes. It's essential to ensure you're getting enough omega-3 by combining all three sources in your diet, whether through food or supplements.

B. Eicosapentaenoic Acid (EPA)

EPA, found in animal products like fatty fish and fish oils, is often used to treat heart disease, heart attacks, depression, and even menopause. All of this and more is done by preventing blood clots, boosting the immune system, and reducing inflammation, pain, and swelling all over the body.

C. Docosahexaenoic Acid (DHA)

DHA can also be found in animal products, including fatty fish and fish oils, as well as meat, eggs, and dairy products. As one of the most important omega-3 fatty acids, it is an important part of the structure of our brains, parts of our eyes, and other parts of our bodies. DHA helps the brain's nervous system work better by keeping membranes healthy and making it easier for brain cells to talk to each other. EPA and DHA are both important for the development of embryos and for healthy aging. Also, they are both precursors to many metabolites that act as lipid mediators. This has led researchers to look into the role of omega-3 supplements as a way to treat a number of diseases.

The Relationship Between Omega-3 Fatty Acids and Anxiety

When compared to other systems, our central nervous system, which includes our brain and spinal cord, has a larger concentration of fat cells. As previously said, DHA is one of the primary types of polyunsaturated fatty acids that comprise our brains and contribute to the proper functioning of our nervous systems. Omega-3 helps fight anxiety by preventing inflammation and boosting the production and maintenance of dopamine.

Inflammation Prevention

Omega-3 fatty acids have been shown to have neuroprotective properties against brain disorders. It protects our brain in part by reducing neuroinflammation. The brain, like other organs, is extremely vulnerable to inflammation. In reality, it is a key part of the way anxiety disorders work and can be treated to make symptoms less severe. Omega-3 and its metabolites act as signaling molecules that stop the immune system from responding in a way that causes unnecessary inflammation.

Dopamine Production and Maintenance

The amygdala (the brain's emotion center), the hippocampus (involved with learning and emotions), and the prefrontal cortex are all linked to anxiety (coordinating complex behavior). Neurotransmitters and/or their related receptors can change in these three parts of the brain, which can lead to big changes in mood. Dopamine, a neurotransmitter, is known to have a key role in anxiety modulation.

Dopamine, sometimes known as a *"feel-good"* neurotransmitter, acts on our brain to influence levels of learning, pleasure, and motivation. Dopamine and its receptors (D1 and D2) are key to how the brain controls anxiety. According to research, complete dopamine depletion in the brain can directly cause anxiety and depression-like behaviors in humans.

How To Respond

Interestingly, omega-3 influences the concentration of dopamine in our brains. When combined with genetics and the environment, it can make us less likely to get an anxiety disorder. A diet high in DHA, in particular, can affect how our brains make and keep dopamine, improve synaptic connections, and improve brain health.

Finding Your Balance

The importance of omega-3 fatty acids in mental health is becoming increasingly widely recognized in the scientific community. Researchers who have looked into its benefits have found that it can help people with anxiety. It is now well established that eating a diet high in omega-3 fatty acids can improve your general health by reducing inflammation, boosting heart health, and protecting your vision. Making small changes to your diet so that you get a moderate amount of omega-3 fats can help your health and lower your risk of anxiety disorders.

Recognizing The Place Of Vitamins In Your Meals To Curbing Anxiety

Vitamins that help curb or manage anxiety disorders include:

A. Magnesium

According to research, magnesium may help with migraines and depression. Chronic pain and anxiety can both be relieved by it. Many people don't get the right amount of magnesium every day, which causes hypomagnesaemia and makes anxiety-related behaviors worse.

Some foods, like spinach, pumpkin seeds, legumes, bananas, and oats, that are naturally high in magnesium may help you feel calmer. Also, many foods have a good amount of tryptophan, an amino acid that the body turns into serotonin and that may help people relax and feel less anxious.

B. B6 vitamin

Getting enough vitamin B6 from food is a key part of helping the body deal with stress and anxiety. More vitamin B6 consumption among women lowers the risk of anxiety, sadness, and panic attacks. For people who are under a lot of stress, magnesium and vitamin B6 work better together.

C. Iron & Vitamin C

Anxiety and depression are known to be exacerbated by low iron. Low iron status is more prevalent in women, who are more likely to experience anxiety.

Heme iron, which comes from red meat and other animal products, and non-heme iron are the two forms of iron that can be found in food (from spinach, legumes, and dried fruit). High-quality protein sources have more iron and make the neurotransmitters dopamine and serotonin, which can improve mental health.

Encourage customers to eat vitamin C-rich foods like citrus, tomatoes, or peppers with non-heme iron at mealtime for improved absorption. These foods also possess anti-inflammatory and cell-protective antioxidant effects.

The Effect Of Caffeine And Sugar On Anxiety

Caffeine and sugar are both stimulants that can affect anxiety levels. Caffeine, a stimulant found in coffee, tea, chocolate, and some medications, can increase feelings of nervousness, jitteriness, and restlessness. High levels of caffeine intake can also lead to insomnia and disrupt sleep patterns, which can exacerbate anxiety symptoms.

Sugar, on the other hand, can also cause a spike in blood sugar levels and then a crash, leading to feelings of irritability, fatigue and mood swings, which can also exacerbate anxiety symptoms. Consuming a diet high in sugar can also disrupt the balance of hormones that regulate stress and anxiety, such as cortisol and serotonin.

It is important to be mindful of your caffeine and sugar intake if you are managing anxiety. It is best to limit or avoid consuming high amounts of caffeine and sugar, and to opt for healthier dietary choices that can support overall well-being and help to manage anxiety symptoms.

Foods That Can Either Alleviate Or Worsen Anxiety

According to studies, some foods help us feel calmer, while others can work as stimulants - at least momentarily. If you suffer from anxiety or panic attacks as a result of stress, making dietary changes may provide anxiety alleviation.

Stress defines the numerous obligations and pressures that we all face on a daily basis. Physical, mental, emotional, or biological stress can all exist. Almost anything you come upon can generate stress.

Anxiety is a symptom or indicator of stress. Rather than life's tragedies or disasters, it is typically the constant interruptions, difficulties, and struggles that produce worry. Listening to a phone ring continually, hearing a new baby's cries, or fretting about paying debts, for example, can generate stress which leads to anxiety.

Chronic anxiety occurs when you are anxious for several days or weeks. The issue with chronic anxiety is that it can lead to long-term health consequences. Even though there are no quick fixes, you can lessen the effects by eating foods that raise or lower certain chemicals in your body.

Some foods relieve anxiety and have a relaxing impact on the body, whereas others cause anxiety after eating.

Here are a few ideas:

- Eat complex carbohydrates, which increase the soothing brain chemical serotonin. Instead of sugary snacks or beverages, choose whole-grain breads and cereals.
- Consume protein at breakfast to maintain energy levels and blood glucose levels.
- Limit or avoid alcohol and caffeine, which create post-meal anxiety. Both have an impact on your sleep and can create agitation.
- Keep hydrated. Dehydration can alter your mood.

Consider including the following foods in your diet to improve your mood:

- Chocolate
- Folate and other vitamin b foods
- Low-glycemic foods
- Magnesium
- Omega-3 fatty acids
- Tryptophan

In addition, consider including zinc-rich foods in your diet. According to research, oysters, cashews, liver, beef, and egg yolks have been linked to reduced anxiety.

A study published in the August 2015 issue of the journal Psychiatry Research found a link between probiotic diets and less social anxiety. Pickles, sauerkraut, and kefir are probiotic foods. In 2017, the journal Annals of General Psychiatry published a new study that linked probiotics to better symptoms of major depressive disorder. This is likely because probiotics reduce inflammation in the body or make more of the calming brain chemical serotonin. Anxiety and depression may be connected.

Check out the five items to add to your diet to raise your mood and the four meals to avoid since they can increase stress and perhaps induce a melancholy mood.

Five (5) Meals To Add To Your Diet

A. Turkey And Tryptophan-Rich Foods

Some studies believe that tryptophan can help reduce stress because it helps your brain create feel-good chemicals. Tryptophan is a precursor to serotonin, and serotonin, a neurotransmitter, helps you feel peaceful.

Tryptophan can be found in a range of foods, including turkey, chicken, bananas, milk, oats, cheese, soy, almonds, peanut butter, and sesame seeds. There is some debate about whether or not tryptophan in food crosses the blood-brain barrier. If it doesn't, then the effect may be small.

B. Beef And Foods High In Vitamin B

Several studies have found a link between the B vitamins, especially thiamine, or vitamin B1, and mood. Some people experience depression when they are deficient in B vitamins such as folic acid and B12. To combat anxiety, take a vitamin B pill or eat foods high in B vitamins. Beef, pig, chicken, leafy greens, legumes, oranges and other citrus fruits, grains, almonds, and eggs are among the foods that can aid with anxiety.

C. Complex carbohydrates

Carbohydrates also boost serotonin synthesis in the brain. When it comes to mood-lifting carbs, experts recommend whole grains like whole-wheat bread or brown rice over processed options like sugar, sweets, or even white bread and white rice. Whole grains take longer to digest and release sugar slowly into the bloodstream. Processed carbs may give you a burst of energy at first, but this is often followed by a spike in insulin, which quickly lowers your blood sugar and makes you feel tired.

D. Omega-3-Rich Foods

Omega-3 fatty acids (EPA and DHA), which are found in fatty fish like salmon, tuna, lake trout, herring, mackerel, anchovies, and sardines, have been shown to be uplifting and improve mood. According to several studies, individuals who took omega-3 fatty acids together with their prescription antidepressants improved better than those who only took antidepressants. Omega-3 fatty acids may lessen the risk of heart disease.

E. Consume Greek yogurt and high-protein foods

Protein stimulates the creation of the brain chemicals norepinephrine and dopamine, both of which are neurotransmitters that convey impulses between nerve cells and, like serotonin, are neurotransmitters. Higher levels of norepinephrine and dopamine have been shown to improve mental energy, alertness, and reaction time. Greek yogurt, fish, meat, cheese, eggs, almonds, beans, soy, and lentils are all high in protein. Combining complex carbohydrates and protein and spreading your meals throughout the day is ideal for mood enhancement.

Five (5) Meals to avoid in your diet

F. Caffeinated beverages including coffee

Some people drink coffee and other caffeine-containing beverages (tea, cola, and hot chocolate) to make them feel more energized. The problem is that people often use caffeine, sugar, and other foods to get a boost of energy. While sugar binges may provide a short boost of serotonin, coffee suppresses serotonin levels in the brain. When serotonin levels are low, you may experience depression and irritability. Caffeine is also a diuretic, meaning it causes you to go to the bathroom more frequently. Dehydration, even minor dehydration, can lead to sadness. Caffeine might also keep you awake, causing worry and anxiety. Remember that in order to be in a good mood, you must get enough sleep.

G. Candy And Sweets

Of course, nearly everyone enjoys desserts. Sweets, especially those containing table sugar, honey, and corn syrup, can also make us feel better— but only for a short time. Here's why: Sugar is readily absorbed into the bloodstream. The absorption produces an initial spike of energy. However, that rush fades when the body increases insulin synthesis to eliminate the sugar from your system. As a result, you're exhausted and depleted.

H. Alcohol

Some people consume alcohol to alleviate stress and anxiety. Unfortunately, the happy mood is fleeting, for it can cause mood swings. Alcohol is depressing in the long run. Alcohol, like caffeine, is a diuretic, and staying hydrated is crucial for a variety of reasons, including mood. If you must drink, do it in moderation. A 6-ounce glass of wine at supper is generally OK. However, you don't want to be a heavy drinker, consuming many bottles with your dinner.

I. Hot Dogs And Processed Foods

Could consuming processed meals like hot dogs, sausage, pies, and cakes cause anxiety? A diet high in processed and fatty foods, according to London researchers, increases the risk of depression. People who ate mostly fried food, processed meat, high-fat dairy items, and sugary desserts had a 58 percent higher risk of melancholy than those who ate "whole" foods like fish and vegetables, according to the study.

Designing A Healthy Meal Plan For Managing Anxiety

Designing a healthy meal plan for managing anxiety involves incorporating nutrient-dense foods that have been shown to have a positive impact on mood and mental health. These include:

- Omega-3 fatty acids: Found in fatty fish such as salmon, mackerel, and sardines, as well as in flaxseeds, chia seeds, and walnuts. These essential fatty acids have anti-inflammatory properties and have been shown to improve mood and reduce symptoms of anxiety.
- Complex carbohydrates: Whole grains, fruits, and vegetables provide essential vitamins and minerals, as well as fiber which can help regulate blood sugar levels, helping to prevent mood swings and feelings of anxiety.
- Protein: Eating adequate amounts of lean protein, such as chicken, fish, turkey, and legumes, can help to balance blood sugar levels and provide the building blocks for neurotransmitters, which play a crucial role in mood regulation.
- Avoid or minimize the intake of caffeine and sugar as they can increase anxiety symptoms.

A healthy meal plan should also include a variety of fruits, vegetables, whole grains, lean protein sources and healthy fats to ensure that you are getting all the essential nutrients your body needs to function properly.

It is important to consult a healthcare professional or a registered dietitian for personalized advice and a personalized meal plan.

Best Supplements To Managing Your Anxiety

Anxiety is a widespread mental health issue. In actuality, almost 33% of people will suffer from an anxiety disorder at some point in their lives.

Generalized Anxiety Disorder (GAD), Panic disorder with or without agoraphobia, Social anxiety disorder (SAD), particular phobias, and separation anxiety disorder are examples of anxiety disorders.

Psychological therapies, such as cognitive behavior therapy, or pharmaceuticals are frequently used in treatment.

But research shows that people with anxiety problems may also benefit from making changes to their diet and taking certain vitamins, minerals, and other supplements.

The following criteria were used to choose the supplements in this list:

- Efficacy: Current study demonstrates that the main elements are both safe and efficient.
- Brand reputation: The supplements are made by trustworthy companies that employ independent research.
- Quality: High-quality components are prioritized in the supplements.

The top 10 supplements for anxiety are shown below:

A. Pure Encapsulations Magnesium Glycinate

Magnesium is a necessary mineral that is vital in the body's stress response.

Furthermore, evidence suggests that magnesium supplements may be beneficial for anxiety sufferers, and that they are generally safe and well tolerated.

For example, a 2017 evaluation of 18 studies indicated that, despite the low quality of existing research, magnesium supplements are likely to aid people suffering from anxiety.

In a 2017 study of 112 people with depression, it was found that taking 248 milligrams (mg) of elemental magnesium supplements every day for 6 weeks made depression and anxiety much less severe than in a control group.

Pure Encapsulations Magnesium Glycinate is a type of magnesium that is very easy to absorb and is great for people with anxiety.

The United States Pharmacopeia (USP), a non-profit group that sets high standards for the identification, quality, and purity of dietary supplements, has approved the supplements.

Pure Encapsulations supplements are tested by third-party labs and do not contain gluten or GMOs.

Every capsule contains 120 milligrams of magnesium.

B. Saffron 50mg Veg Capsules from NOW Foods.

Saffron is a brilliantly colored spice with culinary and medical applications. It's high in antioxidants and may be especially good for people who suffer from anxiety when taken as a supplement.

A 2018 meta-analysis of 100 studies discovered that saffron supplements helped lower anxiety. Some of the studies that were part of the analysis showed that saffron therapy had the same effects on anxiety as the anti-anxiety drug fluoxetine.

Similarly, a 2016 study of 60 individuals with depression and anxiety discovered that taking 100 mg of saffron per day for 12 weeks dramatically reduced anxiety symptoms when compared to a placebo. The subjects tolerated the supplement well, too.

On the other hand, pregnant women should talk to their doctors because there isn't much evidence that saffron supplements don't cause uterine contractions.

NOW Foods Saffron is a wonderful choice because the supplements are non-GMO, vegan, and gluten-free, and they are potency and purity tested by a third party.

Each capsule contains 50 mg of saffron and is recommended to be taken twice a day or as prescribed by your healthcare practitioner.

C. 5000 IU MegaFood Vitamin D3.

Many people don't have enough of this fat-soluble mineral, which is important for brain function and mood control, or they don't have enough of it.

According to research, vitamin D insufficiency or inadequacy is especially common among patients with mental health concerns, such as anxiety disorders.

Furthermore, evidence indicates that taking large levels of vitamin D may be useful in reducing the severity of anxiety symptoms in patients suffering from anxiety disorders, including GAD.

A 2020 study of 106 depressed adults found that taking 1,600 IU of vitamin D per day for 6 months resulted in significant reductions in anxiety symptoms when compared to a control group.

MegaFood Vitamin D3, which contains vitamin D and vitamin K, is one of the best vitamin D supplements for anxiety.

These nutrients work together in the body to help maintain healthy vitamin K levels and promote heart and bone health.

In just one capsule, this supplement provides 5,000 IU of vitamin D and 100% of the Daily Value for vitamin K. As a result, it's a fantastic option for persons who are deficient in vitamin D.

Keep in mind that, while larger dose vitamin D supplements may be required to cure deficiency, a supplement containing 1,000-2,000 IU per day may be more appropriate for persons who just want to maintain healthy vitamin D levels.

Your healthcare expert can evaluate your vitamin D levels and propose the best vitamin D dose for you.

D. Chamomile from Nature's Way.

Chamomile is a herb with relaxing qualities. While it is more usually ingested as a tea, chamomile pills may be beneficial for persons who suffer from anxiety.

According to study, chamomile possesses anti-anxiety and antidepressant qualities.

In one study of 93 people with moderate to severe GAD, daily treatment with 1,500 mg of pharmaceutical-grade chamomile extract for 26 weeks significantly reduced anxiety symptoms compared to a placebo.

Nature's Way Chamomile is a wonderful choice because it is gluten-free and TRU-ID certified, which is a certification scheme that uses DNA testing on components and finished goods to prevent adulteration.

There are 440 mg of chamomile flower and 250 mg of chamomile extract in each serving.

But people who are pregnant or allergic to similar plants like ragweed, chrysanthemums, marigolds, or daisies shouldn't take chamomile supplements because they might not be safe.

Also, chamomile supplements may interact with some medicines, especially those used to treat anxiety. Before taking chamomile supplements, you should talk to your doctor.

E. L-Theanine from Integrative Therapeutics

L-theanine is an amino acid naturally found in green tea. It has been found to help relieve stress and calm anxiety when taken as a supplement.

A 2020 review of nine studies found that taking between 200 and 400 mg of L-theanine per day may help people who are in stressful situations feel less stressed and anxious.

L-theanine supplements have also been shown to help people with schizophrenia or schizoaffective disorder, as well as those with major depressive disorder, by reducing anxiety symptoms.

Integrative Therapeutics L-Theanine is a good choice because the company checks the quality, purity, and effectiveness of both the raw materials and the finished products.

Each serving of two capsules contains 200 mg of L-theanine.

F. Pro Omega 2000 mg from Nordic Naturals

Omega-3 fats have potent anti-inflammatory properties and may be beneficial to people who suffer from anxiety.

A 2018 review of 19 trials showed that taking omega-3 fatty acid supplements made anxiety symptoms much less severe than in control groups.

The analysis did note, though, that significant anti-anxiety effects were only seen in studies that used at least 2,000 mg of omega-3s per day.

Nordic Naturals is well known for producing high-quality omega-3 supplements.

The Nordic Naturals Pro Omega supplement, in particular, is a fantastic alternative for those who suffer from anxiety because it contains 2,000 mg of omega-3s in every two softgels.

On the Nordic Naturals website, each supplement has a "certificate of analysis," which shows that it has been tested for quality and purity and that it meets standards and specifications.

G. Quicksilver Scientific Liposomal Vitamin C.

Vitamin C is a nutrient that acts as a powerful antioxidant in the body, and researchers believe it may help people with neuropsychological disorders, such as anxiety, combat damage caused by oxidative stress.

Furthermore, some studies have shown that vitamin C supplementation can help those who are anxious.

For example, in one study of 42 high school students, taking 500 mg of vitamin C per day for 14 days increased blood vitamin C levels while decreasing anxiety levels.

Adults and women with diabetes who take vitamin C supplements have also been shown to feel less anxious.

Per teaspoon of Quicksilver Scientific Liposomal Vitamin C, you get 1,000 mg of highly absorbable vitamin C (5 mL).

The supplement has liposomal vitamin C, which is a type of vitamin C that is wrapped in tiny lipid spheres and has been shown to be more accessible than vitamin C that is not wrapped in lipid spheres.

This vitamin C supplement comes in a liquid form, which makes it a great choice for people who can't or don't want to take pills.

H. Pure Encapsulations Curcumin 500 with Bioperine.

Curcumin is a polyphenol molecule that is found in turmeric. It has been shown to have anti-inflammatory, antioxidant, antidepressant, and anti-anxiety effects.

In a 2017 study of 123 people with severe depression, those given 500-1,000 mg of curcumin or 500 mg of curcumin combined with 30 mg of saffron per day for 12 weeks improved their anxiety symptoms more than those given a placebo.

Curcumin has also been demonstrated to alleviate anxiety in people with diabetes, obesity, and depression.

Pure Encapsulations Curcumin 500 with Bioperine is one of the best curcumin supplements because each capsule has 500 mg of curcumin and Bioperine, an extract of black pepper that makes it much easier for the body to absorb curcumin.

I. Charlotte's Web 25MG CBD Oil Liquid Capsules

Cannabidiol (CBD) is a popular natural treatment for many health problems, such as anxiety.

Evidence suggests that CBD, in doses ranging from 300 to 600 mg, may help reduce anxiety in those suffering from SAD as well as in those who do not suffer from anxiety disorders.

Furthermore, a recent evaluation of 25 studies discovered that CBD may help lower anxiety in people suffering from SAD. But the researchers did say that many of the studies were not very good, which shows that more good research is needed.

Charlotte's Web is a CBD brand that healthcare professionals trust since the firm is dedicated to keeping customers safe and educated.

Charlotte's Web offers an analysis certificate for each of its items. This documentation informs the consumer of the amount of cannabinoids present in the products, as well as the amounts of pesticides, heavy metals, and tetrahydrocannabinol (THC).

Charlotte's Web 25-milligram CBD oil liquid capsules are a handy way to take CBD, with each capsule containing 25 milligrams of CBD.

It's important to remember that this dose is much lower than those that have been shown to help with anxiety in scientific studies. Before beginning CBD use, consult with your healthcare provider to determine the best dosage for you.

J. Multivitamins

According to research, multivitamin supplements may help alleviate anxiety symptoms.

For instance, one study found that young adults who took a multivitamin with B vitamins, vitamin C, calcium, magnesium, and zinc for 30 days had much less anxiety.

Also, an older review of eight studies found that healthy people who took multivitamin and multimineral supplements for at least 28 days felt less stressed and anxious.

The review also discovered that supplements with high doses of B vitamins may be more effective than those with low doses of B vitamins.

Remember that multivitamins aren't one-size-fits-all, and some multivitamins may be inappropriate for certain people due to nutrient demands varying with age, gender, and overall health.

For example, younger women may benefit from getting more iron in their diet, while men and women who have gone through menopause tend to need less iron.

Before you start taking multivitamins to treat your anxiety, talk to your doctor. He or she can help you choose a product that is right for your needs.

How To Make The Choice That Fits You

If you're thinking about using supplements to help with anxiety, you should first consult with your doctor.

Not all supplements are safe or acceptable for those who suffer from anxiety, especially if you are already taking medication.

Be wary of supplement mixtures that claim to treat or cure anxiety.

Although some supplements have been found to help alleviate anxiety symptoms, other interventions such as therapy, dietary and lifestyle changes, and medication may be more beneficial.

When shopping for supplements, only buy from reputed producers.

Examine supplements that have been certified by third-party organizations such as NSF International and USP. These organizations test supplements for potency, contaminants, and other factors to guarantee that customers receive a safe and high-quality product.

In Summary

Anxiety is a common mental health problem. It may interfere with certain people's regular activities.

Anxiety disorders, fortunately, can be treated with counseling, medication, and dietary changes, including supplements.

Certain nutritional supplements, such as magnesium, vitamin D, saffron, omega-3s, chamomile, L-theanine, vitamin C, curcumin, CBD, and multivitamins, have been shown in studies to help relieve anxiety symptoms.

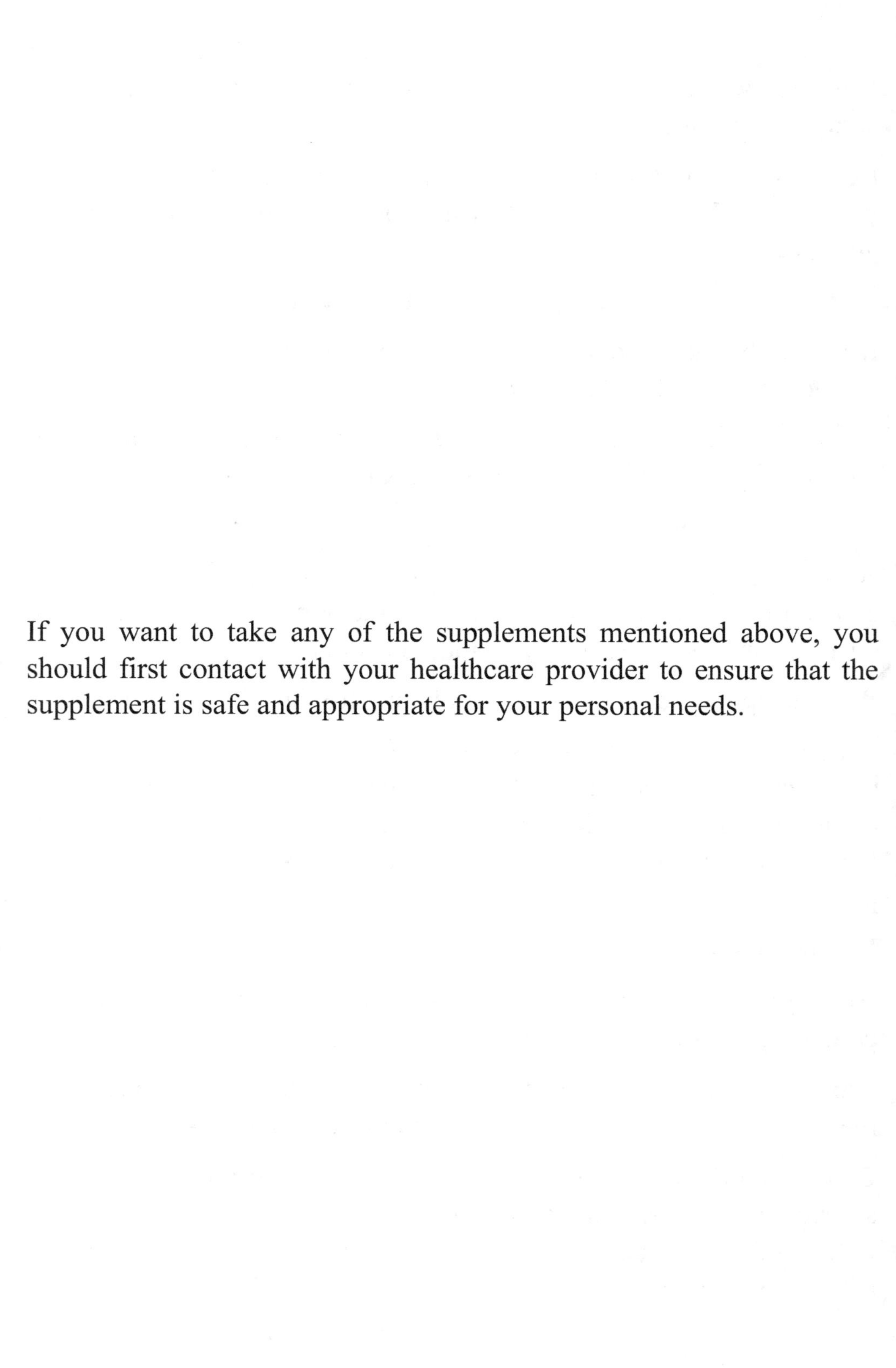

If you want to take any of the supplements mentioned above, you should first contact with your healthcare provider to ensure that the supplement is safe and appropriate for your personal needs.

MEDICATIONS AND THERAPY OPTIONS FOR TREATING ANXIETY

There are several medications and therapy options available for treating anxiety. Some common medications used to treat anxiety include selective serotonin reuptake inhibitors (SSRIs), serotonin-norepinephrine reuptake inhibitors (SNRIs), and benzodiazepines. SSRIs and SNRIs are types of antidepressants that work by increasing the levels of certain chemicals in the brain, such as serotonin and norepinephrine, which can help to improve mood and reduce anxiety. Benzodiazepines are a type of sedative that can help to reduce anxiety symptoms quickly, but they are typically used on a short-term basis.

In addition to medication, therapy is also an effective treatment option for anxiety. The most common types of therapy used to treat anxiety include Cognitive Behavioral Therapy (CBT), exposure therapy, and Acceptance and Commitment Therapy (ACT).

CBT is a type of therapy that helps individuals to identify and change negative thoughts and beliefs that contribute to their anxiety. The therapist will work with the individual to understand the connections between their thoughts, feelings and behaviors and teach them new ways of thinking and behaving that can help to reduce their anxiety.

Exposure therapy is a type of therapy that involves gradually exposing the individual to the source of their anxiety in a controlled environment. This can help the individual to learn that their fear or anxiety is not as dangerous as they once thought, and that they can cope with it.

ACT is a mindfulness-based therapy that helps individuals to accept their thoughts and feelings without trying to change them. This can help to reduce the struggle and suffering caused by anxiety, and allow individuals to engage in the activities that they value in their life.

It is important to note that different people may respond differently to different treatments, and it may take some time to find the right combination of therapy and medication that works best for an individual. It is important to work closely with a mental health professional to determine the most appropriate treatment plan.

Understanding The Different Types Of Medications Used To Treat Anxiety Disorders

Medications used to treat anxiety disorders can be broadly categorized into several classes, including:

A. **Anti-anxiety medications**: These medications help to reduce feelings of anxiety and nervousness. Examples include benzodiazepines (such as diazepam, alprazolam, lorazepam), buspirone, and beta-blockers.

B. **Antidepressants**: Certain types of antidepressants, such as selective serotonin reuptake inhibitors (SSRIs), have been found to be effective in treating anxiety disorders. Examples include fluoxetine, sertraline, and paroxetine.

C. **Beta-blockers**: These medications are typically used to treat high blood pressure, but they can also help to reduce physical symptoms of anxiety such as a fast heartbeat, sweating, and shaking.

D. **Tricyclic antidepressants**: These medications were originally developed to treat depression, but some can also be effective for anxiety. Examples include imipramine and amitriptyline.

NB: It is important to note that medications alone are not usually a long-term solution for anxiety disorders, and they are often best used in conjunction with therapy, such as cognitive-behavioral therapy (CBT). Additionally, medications may have side effects and should be used under the supervision of a healthcare professional.

Anxiety symptoms can be treated with a variety of medications. The four major classes of medicines for anxiety disorders, according to the Anxiety and Depression Association of America (ADAA), are:

A. Selective Serotonin Reuptake Inhibitors (SSRI)

Selective serotonin reuptake inhibitors (SSRIs) are a type of antidepressant that is frequently used.

They are usually used along with a talking therapy like cognitive behavioral therapy (CBT) to treat depression, especially when it is severe or lasts for a long time.

Because they have fewer negative effects than most other types of antidepressants, SSRIs are usually the first choice of treatment for depression.

In addition to treating depression, SSRIs can be used to treat a variety of other mental health problems, such as:

- Generalized Anxiety Disorder (GAD)
- Obsessive Compulsive Disorder (OCD)
- Panic Disorder
- Severe phobias, such as agoraphobia and social phobia
- Bulimia
- Post-Traumatic Stress Disorder (PTSD)

SSRIs are also used to treat premenstrual syndrome (PMS), fibromyalgia, and irritable bowel syndrome (IBS), among other conditions. They are occasionally administered to treat pain.

The Action Mechanism of SSRIs

SSRIs are supposed to act by boosting serotonin levels in the brain.

Serotonin is a type of neurotransmitter (a messenger chemical that carries signals between nerve cells in the brain). It is supposed to have a positive effect on mood, emotion, and sleep.

Serotonin is frequently reabsorbed by nerve cells after conveying a message (known as "reuptake"). SSRIs function by inhibiting ("blocking") reuptake, which means that more serotonin is available to send messages between neighboring nerve cells.

It would be too simple to say that depression and other mental health problems are caused by low serotonin levels, but raising serotonin levels can help relieve symptoms and make people more receptive to other treatments, like cognitive-behavioral therapy (CBT).

Dosages And Treatment Duration

SSRIs are often administered as tablets. When you are given them, you will start with the lowest dose that will make your symptoms better.

SSRIs are typically administered for 2–4 weeks before any benefit is felt. At first, you may have some minor side effects, but it is very important that you keep taking the medicine. These effects often fade soon.

If you've been taking an SSRI for 4 to 6 weeks and haven't noticed any improvement, consult your doctor or a mental health specialist. They may advise you to increase your dose or try a different antidepressant.

Normal treatment should last at least 6 months after you feel better, but sometimes longer treatments are needed, and people who have problems that keep coming back may be told to keep taking them forever.

Note the following

SSRIs are not appropriate for everyone. Due to the higher risk of serious side effects, they are usually not recommended for people under 18 or who are pregnant or breastfeeding. But if the benefits of therapy are thought to be greater than the risks, an exception may be made.

If you have diabetes, epilepsy, or a kidney disease, for example, you should be careful when taking SSRIs.

Some SSRIs can have unpredictable interactions with other medications, including over-the-counter pain relievers and herbal therapies like St. John's wort. Always read the information booklet that comes with your SSRI medication to see if there are any other medications that you should avoid.

Adverse Consequences

When using SSRIs, most people will only encounter a few minor adverse effects. These can be difficult at first, but they usually improve with time.

Common SSRI side effects include:

- Feeling agitated, shaky or anxious
- Diarrhea
- Feeling of being sick
- Dizziness
- Blurred vision
- Loss of libido (reduced sex drive)
- Difficulty achieving orgasm during sex or masturbation
- In men, difficulty obtaining or maintaining an erection (erectile dysfunction)

When you first start taking an SSRI, you should see your doctor every few weeks to talk about how well the drug is working. You can also talk to your doctor at any time if you have side effects that bother you or keep coming back.

SSRI classifications

In the United Kingdom, the following SSRIs are currently prescribed:

- citalopram (Cipramil)
- dapoxetine (Priligy)
- escitalopram (Cipralex)
- fluoxetine (Prozac or Oxactin)
- fluvoxamine (Faverin)
- Sertraline (Lustral) with paroxetine (Seroxat) (Brintellix)

B. Serotonin-Norepinephrine Reuptake Inhibitors (SNRI)

Serotonin and norepinephrine reuptake inhibitors (SNRIs) are a type of drug used to treat depression. SNRIs are also sometimes used to treat anxiety disorders and long-term (chronic) pain, particularly nerve pain. If you suffer from chronic pain in addition to depression, SNRIs may be beneficial.

How SNRIs Function

SNRIs help with depression by changing the chemicals that brain cells use to talk to each other. These chemicals are called neurotransmitters. SNRIs, like most antidepressants, help treat depression by causing changes in brain chemistry and communication in brain nerve cell circuits known to influence mood.

SNRIs inhibit the brain's reabsorption (reuptake) of the neurotransmitters serotonin and norepinephrine.

SNRIs have been licensed for the treatment of depression.

The Food and Drug Administration (FDA) has approved the following SNRIs for the treatment of depression:

- Desvenlafaxine (Pristiq)
- Duloxetine (Cymbalta) is also licensed for the treatment of anxiety and some types of chronic pain.
- Levomilnacipran (Fetzima)
- Venlafaxine (Effexor XR) is also licensed to treat anxiety and panic disorders.

Precautions And Side Effects

All SNRIs act in the same way and can have comparable side effects, although some people may not experience any. Side effects are usually minor and disappear after a few weeks of medication. Taking your prescription with food may help you feel less nauseated. Because each SNRI has a different chemical makeup, if you can't tolerate one, you might be able to take another.

The following are the most prevalent SNRI side effects:

- Nausea
- Parched mouth
- Dizziness
- Headache
- Sweating excessively
- Tiredness
- Constipation
- Insomnia
- Sexual function changes, such as decreased sexual desire, difficulties reaching orgasm, or inability to sustain an erection (erectile dysfunction)
- Appetite loss

In most cases, the benefits of antidepressants outweigh the potential adverse effects. Which antidepressant is appropriate for you is determined by a number of factors, including your symptoms and any other medical conditions you may have.

Inquire with your doctor and pharmacist about the most prevalent adverse effects associated with your specific SNRI, and read the patient medication information that comes with the prescription.

Concerns About Safety

Most people are not adversely affected by SNRIs. However, in rare cases, they can be problematic. As an example:

- Venlafaxine, desvenlafaxine, and levomilnacipran can all cause an increase in blood pressure.
- Duloxetine may exacerbate liver issues.

Other issues to discuss with your doctor before using an SNRI are as follows:

A. Drug Interactions: Inform your doctor about any additional prescription or OTC drugs, herbs, or supplements you're using. Some antidepressants can have very bad side effects if they are taken with certain drugs or natural substances. SNRIs, for example, may raise your risk of bleeding, particularly if you are also taking other medications that increase your risk of bleeding, such as ibuprofen (Advil, Motrin IB, and others), aspirin, warfarin (Coumadin, Jantoven), and other blood thinners.

B. Serotonin Syndrome: Serotonin syndrome can arise in rare cases when you take antidepressants that cause serotonin levels in your body to rise. This is particularly common when two serotonin-raising drugs, such as antidepressants, pain or headache treatments, or St. John's wort, are combined.

Anxiety, agitation, high fever, sweating, confusion, tremors, restlessness, loss of coordination, substantial variations in blood pressure, and a rapid heart rate are signs and symptoms of serotonin syndrome.

If you have any of these symptoms, get emergency medical attention.

C. Pregnancy And Antidepressants: Discuss the dangers and benefits of specific antidepressants with your doctor. Some antidepressants can be harmful to your infant if used during pregnancy or while breastfeeding. If you're taking an antidepressant and thinking about becoming pregnant, talk to your doctor about the dangers. Do not discontinue your medicine without first consulting your doctor, as doing so may endanger your health.

Antidepressants And The Risk Of Suicide

Even though most antidepressants are safe, the FDA requires that they all have black box warnings, which are the strongest prescription warnings. Children, teenagers, and young adults under the age of 25 may experience an increase in suicidal thoughts or behavior when taking antidepressants, particularly in the first few weeks or when the dose is altered.

People who take antidepressants should always be watched for signs of getting worse or acting strange. If you or someone you know has had suicidal thoughts while taking an antidepressant, contact your doctor or seek emergency care right away.

Keep in mind that antidepressants, by increasing mood, are more likely to minimize suicide risk in the long run.

When To Stop Treatment With SNRIs

SNRIs are not thought to be addictive. However, suddenly discontinuing antidepressant treatment or missing several doses may result in withdrawal symptoms. This is known as "discontinuation syndrome." SNRIs like venlafaxine and desvenlafaxine may cause withdrawal-like symptoms more often, but they can happen with any SNRI. Work with your doctor to reduce your dose gradually and carefully.

Symptoms of withdrawal can include:

- Dizziness
- Headache
- Flu-like symptoms include fatigue, chills, and muscle aches.
- Agitation or irritability
- Nausea
- Insomnia or sleeping problems, such as nightmares
- Diarrhea

Choosing The Best Antidepressant

People may have various reactions to the same medication. For example, a specific medicine may work better or worse for you than for someone else. Or, you might have more or less side effects from a particular antidepressant than someone else.

Inherited traits influence how antidepressants affect you. In some situations, if available, the findings of special blood tests may provide information about how your body may react to a specific antidepressant. However, factors other than genetics can influence your response to treatment.

When selecting an antidepressant, your doctor considers your symptoms, any health issues, other medications you are taking, and what has worked in the past for you.

It can take several weeks or longer for an antidepressant to become fully effective and for its initial adverse effects to subside. Your doctor may suggest dose modifications or switching antidepressants, but with time and effort, you and your doctor can discover a drug that works well for you.

C. Tricyclic Antidepressants (TCA)

Tricyclic and tetracyclic antidepressants, commonly known as "cyclic antidepressants," were among the first to be produced. They work, but most of them have been replaced by antidepressants that have fewer side effects. Cyclical antidepressants, on the other hand, may be a good alternative for some people. In certain circumstances, they can alleviate depression after other treatments have failed.

The number of rings in the chemical structure of cyclic antidepressants determines whether they are tricyclic or tetracyclic.

How Cyclic Antidepressants Work

Cyclic antidepressants help people feel better by changing the chemicals (neurotransmitters) that brain cells use to talk to each other. Cyclical antidepressants, like most antidepressants, assist in treating depression by causing changes in brain chemistry and communication in brain nerve cell circuits known to influence mood.

Cyclic antidepressants stop the brain chemicals serotonin and norepinephrine from being taken back up, which raises their levels in the brain. Cyclic antidepressants also affect other chemical messengers, which could cause a wide range of side effects.

Cyclic antidepressants have been licensed for the treatment of depression.

The following tricyclic antidepressants have been approved by the Food and Drug Administration (FDA) for treating depression:

- Amitriptyline
- Amoxapine
- Desipramine (Norpramin)
- Doxepin
- Imipramine (Tofranil)
- Nortriptyline (Pamelor)
- Protriptyline
- Trimipramine
- Maprotiline, a tetracyclic antidepressant, has been approved by the FDA to treat depression.

Other than depression, cyclic antidepressants are sometimes used to treat obsessive-compulsive disorder, anxiety disorders, and nerve-related (neuropathic) pain.

Side Effects And Precautions

Because of the various mechanisms by which cyclic antidepressants function, adverse effects vary from drug to drug. Some side effects may fade over time, while others may prompt you and your doctor to switch medications. Side effects may also be dose-dependent, with greater doses frequently generating more side effects.

Some of the most common potential adverse effects include:

- Drowsiness
- Vision distortion
- Constipation
- Parched mouth
- Drop in blood pressure
- Retention of urine
- Weight reduction
- Sweating excessively
- Tremor

- Sexual issues such as erection trouble, delayed orgasm, or poor sex desire

Note:

Amitriptyline, doxepin, imipramine, and trimipramine are more likely than other tricyclic antidepressants to cause sleepiness. Taking these drugs before bed may be beneficial.

Amitriptyline, doxepin, imipramine, and trimipramine are more likely than other tricyclic antidepressants to cause weight gain.

The side effects of nortriptyline and desipramine tend to be less severe than those of other tricyclic antidepressants.

When taking antidepressants that cause one to sleep, avoid undertaking tasks that need one to be alert, such as driving.

The right antidepressant for you depends on a number of things, such as your symptoms and any other health problems you may have. Inquire with your doctor and pharmacist about the most common adverse effects associated with your specific antidepressant, and read the patient medication information that comes with the prescription.

Safety Concerns

Some tricyclic antidepressants are more likely to induce dangerous adverse effects, such as:

- When the dosage is excessively high, it might cause disorientation or confusion, especially in older adults.
- Heart rate that is too fast or too slow.
- Seizures occur more frequently in those who have seizures.

Other things to talk about with your doctor before starting a cyclic antidepressant:

A. Antidepressants and pregnancy: Talk to your doctor about the risks and benefits of using certain antidepressants during pregnancy. Some antidepressants can be harmful to your infant if used during pregnancy or while breastfeeding. If you're taking an antidepressant and thinking about becoming pregnant, talk to your doctor or a mental health expert about the risks. Don't stop taking your medicine without talking to your doctor first, because doing so could hurt your health.

B. Drug interactions: Tell your doctor about any additional prescription or over-the-counter drugs, herbs, or supplements you're taking if you're taking an antidepressant. When coupled with certain drugs or herbal supplements, some antidepressants might induce serious side effects.

C. Serotonin syndrome: Rarely, an antidepressant can induce excessive serotonin accumulation in your body. Serotonin syndrome is most commonly caused by the combination of two drugs that increase serotonin levels. Other antidepressants, pain relievers, and the natural supplement in this category is St. John's wort.

Serotonin syndrome is marked by anxiety, agitation, a high fever, sweating, confusion, tremors, restlessness, loss of coordination, large changes in blood pressure, and a fast heart rate.

If you notice any of these signs or symptoms, seek medical attention right away.

D. Blood testing and safety: Your doctor may advise you to take blood tests to identify the most effective dose. Some of the negative effects and benefits of cyclic antidepressants are dose dependent. An overdose of cyclic antidepressants can be fatal.

E. Chronic health problems: Cyclic antidepressants can produce complications in those who have specific medical issues. If you have glaucoma, an enlarged prostate, heart issues, diabetes, liver disease, or a history of seizures, consult your doctor about whether a cyclic antidepressant is a good option for you.

Antidepressants And The Risk Of Suicide

Even though most antidepressants are safe, the FDA requires that they all have black box warnings, which are the strongest prescription warnings. Children, teenagers, and young adults under the age of 25 may experience an increase in suicidal thoughts or behavior when taking antidepressants, particularly in the first few weeks or when the dose is altered.

People who take antidepressants should always be watched for signs of getting worse or acting strange. If you or someone you know has had suicidal thoughts while taking an antidepressant, contact your doctor or seek emergency care right away.

Keep in mind that antidepressants, by increasing mood, are more likely to minimize suicide risk in the long run.

When to Discontinue Treatment With Cyclic Antidepressants

Cyclic antidepressants are not addictive. However, suddenly discontinuing antidepressant treatment or missing several doses can result in withdrawal symptoms. Depending on how the medicine works, symptoms may differ. This is known as "discontinuation syndrome." Work with your doctor to reduce your dose gradually and carefully.

Symptoms of withdrawal can include:

- Anger, irritation, or agitation
- Nausea
- Sweating Flu symptoms include chills and muscular aches
- Insomnia
- Lethargy
- Headache

Choosing The Best Antidepressant

People may have various reactions to the same medication. For example, a specific medicine may work better or worse for you than for someone else. Or, you might have more or less side effects from a particular antidepressant than someone else.

Inherited traits may influence how medications affect you. In some cases, if they are available, the results of certain blood tests may show how your body might react to a certain antidepressant. However, factors other than genetics can influence your response to treatment.

When selecting an antidepressant, your doctor considers your symptoms, any health issues, other medications you are taking, and what has previously worked for you.

It can take several weeks or longer for an antidepressant to become fully effective and for its initial adverse effects to subside. Your doctor may suggest dose modifications or switching antidepressants, but with time and effort, you and your doctor can discover a drug that works well for you.

D. Benzodiazepines

Benzodiazepines, sometimes known as "benzos," are a class of drugs known for their sedative and anti-anxiety properties. They can be beneficial in the treatment of anxiety, but they also have some risks and adverse effects that you should be aware of.

These drugs were once the most commonly used anxiety therapies, but there are now newer and often more effective treatments available that do not have many of the same hazards as benzodiazepines. If you suffer from anxiety, learning more about the use of benzodiazepines to treat it will help you decide if this is the best treatment option for you.

How Benzodiazepines Help with Anxiety

Benzodiazepines have an effect on the brain's gamma-aminobutyric acid (GABA) receptors. This activity slows down the central nervous system (CNS), which makes a person feel calm. Benzodiazepines are rather fast-acting, easing symptoms in a short period of time.

They can also be used to treat sleeplessness, which can be a symptom of or a contributing factor to anxiety. Anxiety can make it hard to fall asleep, but not getting enough sleep can also cause or make anxiety symptoms worse.

Anxiety Dosages

Depending on your condition and symptoms, you can take benzodiazepines once a day, more than once a day, or only when you need them. Your doctor may start you on a low dose and gradually increase it if you continue to have symptoms.

The therapeutic dosage varies widely from person to person. It could also depend on how bad the symptoms are and how the person's body works.

Actual Dosage

- Lorazepam (Ativan): 0.5 to 1 mg three to four times per day.
- Klonopin (clonazepam): 0.5 to 1 mg three times daily, with a daily maximum of 20 mg.
- Librium (chlordiazepoxide): 5 to 25 mg three to four times a day, with a daily limit of 100 mg.
- Serax (oxazepam): 10 to 30 mg three to four times a day, with a daily maximum of 120 mg.
- Valium (diazepam): 5 to 25 mg three to four times a day, with a maximum daily dose of 40 mg.
- 0.25 to 1 mg of Xanax (alprazolam) three times per day. The daily maximum dose is 4 mg.

In addition to benzodiazepines, your doctor may suggest psychotherapy to help address your anxiety. According to research, combining drugs and therapy may be the most effective treatment strategy.

Cognitive-behavioral therapy (CBT), a type of therapy, is one of the most commonly utilized treatments to manage anxiety.

Types of Benzodiazepines for Anxiety

Benzodiazepines are commonly used to treat anxiety, panic attacks, and sleeplessness. The following benzodiazepines are used to treat anxiety-related panic disorder or other anxiety disorders:

A. **Xanax (alprazolam):** short-term treatment for anxiety symptoms.

B. **Klonopin (clonazepam):** This medication is used to treat panic disorder and panic attacks.

C. **Valium (diazepam):** This medication may be prescribed during the first phase of treatment for panic disorder.

D. **Ativan (lorazepam):** Used to treat anxiety symptoms associated with other psychiatric illnesses.

E. **Librium (chlordiazepoxide):** This medication can be used to treat anxiety problems as well as alcohol withdrawal symptoms.

Benzodiazepines can also be used to treat things like seizures, muscle spasms, and withdrawal from alcohol or other drugs. They can also be used to treat sleep disturbances and relax patients before surgery.

Precautions When Taking Benzodiazepines

Benzodiazepines should only be used as prescribed by your doctor. Do not raise your dosage without first visiting your doctor. If your doctor has given you a benzodiazepine, don't stop taking it without first talking to him or her. This may result in undesirable withdrawal symptoms or worsen your health and symptoms.

Benzodiazepines are listed as Schedule IV restricted substances in the United States.

Safe Usage

Drowsiness caused by benzodiazepines can impair your ability to drive safely. If you are tired or sleepy, you should avoid driving or using heavy machinery. Benzodiazepines should not be combined with alcohol or other sedatives.

Drug Interactions

Some medications, especially some SSRIs, may change how your body breaks down and gets rid of benzodiazepines. This may result in an increase in the amount of benzodiazepine medicine in your blood. When taking benzodiazepines with SSRIs or other drugs, it is important to follow your doctor's dosing instructions to avoid an increased risk of overdose or unwanted side effects.

Combining benzodiazepines with alcohol or other drugs that slow down the central nervous system (CNS) may make the CNS slow down even more.

These combinations have the potential to be dangerous, increasing the risk of overdose. There have been reports of deaths as a result of these interactions.

This is not an exhaustive list. Your doctor says you should try to avoid other drug interactions and health problems before starting benzodiazepine therapy.

Inform your doctor about any prescriptions, including over-the-counter medications and vitamins. Talk to your doctor or pharmacist before taking any prescription or over-the-counter medicine that has benzodiazepines in it.

Breastfeeding and Pregnancy

When taken during the first trimester of pregnancy, benzodiazepines have been associated with congenital birth abnormalities. They're also found in human breast milk. If you are using benzodiazepines and become pregnant, contact your doctor as soon as possible.

Age

Benzodiazepines should not be used to treat anxiety in children or teenagers. These drugs may produce irritation symptoms rather than feelings of relaxation.

Furthermore, older people may be more susceptible to the effects of benzodiazepines. Because of this, people may be more likely to feel confused and have trouble coordinating their muscles, which can lead to falls, broken bones, or other accidents.

Health Problems

Tell your doctor if you have any of the following conditions before starting benzodiazepine therapy:

- A history of alcoholism or other substance addiction.
- Glaucoma.
- Disease of the kidneys or the liver.
- Seizures in the past.
- Bipolar disorder or depression in the past.
- Suicidal ideation.

If you are suicidal, call the National Suicide Prevention Lifeline at 988 for help and support from a certified counselor. (Call 911 if you or a loved one is in urgent danger.)

Benzodiazepine Side Effects

Drowsiness and poor coordination are the most typical negative effects of benzodiazepine use. When benzodiazepines are taken in low doses for short periods of time, such side effects are usually minimal and may not be visible or bothersome. Other possible adverse effects include:

- Confusion
- Fatigue
- Impaired memory
- Slow Mental processing

When the effects of the medications wear off, the side effects of benzodiazepines fade. When used to treat insomnia, you may feel tired the next day even though you got enough sleep the night before.

Speak with your healthcare professional if any of these or other negative effects persist.

It's also worth mentioning that this class of drugs comes with an FDA black box warning about the serious hazards of abuse, addiction, physical dependency, and withdrawal.

Even when taken at regulated doses, benzodiazepines can cause physical dependence, and sudden discontinuation can result in severe withdrawal symptoms, including seizures.

Risk of Overdose

Benzodiazepines are generally safe and effective when used as prescribed. People have died from taking too many benzodiazepines alone or with alcohol or other drugs. These occurrences have the potential to be fatal.

Overdose symptoms and signs include:

- Extreme Sedation
- Confusion
- Coordination issues
- Reduced reflexes
- Difficulty breathing
- Coma

If a benzodiazepine overdose is suspected, seek emergency medical treatment.

Tolerance, Dependence, and Withdrawal

If you take benzodiazepines for a long time, especially in high doses, your body could become physically dependent on them. They can also be mentally addictive in some people.

Research shows that people who take benzodiazepines for a long time may develop a tolerance, which makes the drugs less effective. If tolerance builds up, you may need to take more benzodiazepines to get the same effects.

If you take benzodiazepines for a long time, your body may get used to them and have withdrawal symptoms if you stop taking them suddenly or take less of them. Among the withdrawal symptoms are:

- Anxiety
- Diarrhea and stomach discomfort.

- Insomnia.
- Muscle Cramps
- Headache
- Reduced concentration
- Fast Breathing
- Tremors
- Seizures

Do not stop or reduce your benzodiazepine prescription without first consulting your doctor. To avoid withdrawal symptoms, you may need to gradually reduce your dosage.

Benzodiazepine Substitutes

Benzodiazepines are strong and work quickly, which makes them a great alternative for acute anxiety attacks that don't last long. However, benzodiazepines are not the only choice for treating anxiety disorders. Antidepressants, beta-blockers, and a medicine called BuSpar are some other medications that may be administered to alleviate anxiety.

Supplements and over-the-counter (OTC) anxiety medications may also be beneficial in some cases. Anxiety can be relieved using herbal treatments such as chamomile, lavender, l-theanine, and valerian.

Antihistamines, such as Benadryl, are sometimes used off-label to treat anxiety symptoms. Cannabidiol (CBD) may potentially provide some relief from anxiety symptoms.

Modifications to one's lifestyle might also help to alleviate anxiety. Getting enough sleep, limiting coffee intake, and engaging in regular exercise can all help keep worry at bay.

Other Anti-Anxiety Medicines

Many other medications may help treat anxiety, but they are normally prescribed only if SSRIs or similar therapies do not work.

Other anxiety drugs include:

E. Beta-Blockers

Beta-blockers are a type of drug that helps moderate your body's fight-or-flight response and lessens its negative effects on your heart. Many people use beta-blockers to address heart diseases like:

- High blood pressure
- Heart failure
- An erratic heartbeat

Doctors can also prescribe beta-blockers for off-label purposes, such as reducing anxiety symptoms. Continue reading to learn more about how beta-blockers affect anxiety and whether they could help you.

How Do Beta-Blockers Function

Beta-blockers are sometimes known as beta-adrenergic blockers. They keep adrenaline, a stress hormone, from interacting with your heart's beta receptors. This keeps adrenaline from making your heart beat faster or harder.

Some beta-blockers relax your blood vessels as well as your heart, which can help lower your blood pressure.

There are numerous beta-blockers available, but some of the most prevalent ones are as follows:

- Acebutolol (Sectral)
- Bisoprolol (Zebeta)
- Carvedilol (Coreg)
- Propranolol (Inderal)
- Atenolol (Tenormin)
- Metoprolol (Lopressor)

All beta-blockers are prescribed off-label to relieve anxiety. Propranolol and atenolol are two beta-blockers that are commonly used to treat anxiety.

Off-label usage of a drug indicates that a drug has been approved by the FDA for one purpose but is being used for another that has not been approved. Because the FDA regulates drug testing and approval, not how doctors use them to treat their patients, a doctor can still prescribe it for this purpose. If your doctor believes it is best for your care, he or she may prescribe an off-label medication.

How Do Beta-Blockers Alleviate Anxiety

Although beta-blockers will not treat the underlying psychological reasons for anxiety, they will help you manage some of your body's physical responses to anxiety, such as:

- Rapid heart rate
- Shaky voice and hands
- Sweating
- Dizziness

You may feel less worried during difficult times if you reduce your body's physical reactions to stress.

Short-term anxiety about specific events, rather than long-term anxiety, is best managed with beta-blockers. For example, if giving a public speech makes you nervous, you can take a beta-blocker beforehand.

The effects of short-term use of propranolol to treat anxiety disorders were found to be similar to those of benzodiazepines in a 2016 review of the available data. This is another type of medicine that is frequently used to treat anxiety and panic disorders. However, benzodiazepines can have a variety of negative effects, and some people are more likely to become reliant on them.

Nonetheless, the same study indicated that beta-blockers were ineffective for social phobias.

Medication affects everyone differently, especially when it comes to addressing mental health disorders like anxiety. What works for one individual might not work at all for another. While taking beta-blockers, you may need other types of therapy to deal with the more psychological parts of your anxiety.

How Do I Take Beta-Blockers for Anxiety?

Both atenolol and propranolol are available as pills. The amount you should take is determined by the type of beta-blocker you are taking as well as your medical history. Never take more than your doctor has prescribed.

You'll probably notice results the first time you take beta-blockers for anxiety, but it may take an hour or two for the entire effect to kick in. During this time, your heart rate will likely slow, making you feel more relaxed.

Depending on how you feel, your doctor may tell you to take a beta-blocker every day or only when you're going to be stressed. Most of the time, beta-blockers are used with other treatments like therapy, changes in lifestyle, and other medicines.

What Are The Possible Consequences

Beta-blockers can have some negative effects, especially when first started.

The following are possible adverse effects:

- Fatigue
- Cold hands and feet
- Headache
- Feeling dizzy or lightheaded
- Depression
- Breathing difficulty
- Vomiting, diarrhea, or constipation

Contact your doctor if you are severely experiencing the following side effects:

- Low blood sugar levels
- Asthma attack
- Irregular/slow heart beat

- Weight gain that is accompanied with edema and fluid retention.

If you have minor side effects, you shouldn't stop taking the beta-blocker without talking to your doctor first. If you take beta-blockers on a regular basis, you may experience severe withdrawal symptoms if you suddenly stop taking them.

Some people may experience anxiety symptoms as a result of beta-blocker side effects. If you think that beta-blockers are making your anxiety worse, you should talk to your doctor right away.

Who Should Avoid Beta-Blockers?

While beta-blockers are generally safe, they should not be used by some patients.

Consult your doctor before using beta-blockers if you have the following symptoms:

- Low blood sugar levels
- Very slow heart-beat rate
- Heart failure, at the final stage
- Asthma

If you have any of these diseases or symptoms, you might still be able to take beta-blockers, but you should talk to your doctor about the risks and benefits.

Beta-blockers can also cause problems with other medicines used to treat heart diseases and depression. Tell your doctor about all the medicines, supplements, and vitamins you take.

In conclusion

Beta-blockers can help some people with anxiety manage their symptoms. It has been shown to be an effective way to treat short-term anxiety, especially before something stressful. Beta-blockers, on the other hand, aren't as effective for long-term treatment.

Speak with your doctor if you want to try beta-blockers for anxiety management. They can advise you on the best treatment plan for your specific symptoms.

F. Monoamine Oxidase Inhibitors (MAOIs)

MAOIs are antidepressant medications. According to the 2021 study, doctors began prescribing MAOIs in the 1950s, making them the earliest type of antidepressant.

Nowadays, doctors usually only prescribe this type of medication when other medications have failed. This is because people who take MAOIs have to be very careful about what they eat and because these drugs can have serious side effects.

How do they function?

MAOIs disrupt the chemical balance in the brain. These chemicals are known as neurotransmitters, and they are required for proper brain function.

MAOIs inhibit the enzyme monoamine oxidase, which breaks down neurotransmitters in the brain. This type of medication raises the levels of these neurotransmitters.

According to a 2020 study, while scientists are unsure about the underlying causes of depression, changes in serotonin levels appear to have had a significant impact.

Serotonin is just one of many neurotransmitters, and scientists think that changes in the levels of other neurotransmitters may be linked to depression.

These are some examples:

- Brain-derived neurotrophic factor
- Norepinephrine
- Dopamine
- Glutamate

What Exactly Are Monoamine Oxidases and What Are They Used For?

Monoamine oxidases are enzymes that degrade specific neurotransmitters.

Monoamine oxidases are classified into two types: MAO-A and MAO-B. The following neurotransmitters are broken down by both types:

- Norepinephrine
- Dopamine
- Tyramine
- Tryptamine

The most important enzyme in the breakdown of serotonin is epinephrine (MAO-A).

As MAOIs inhibit this enzyme, serotonin, norepinephrine, and dopamine levels rise. When this happens in the brain of someone suffering from depression, their symptoms may improve.

What MAOIs Are There?

This category includes a variety of drugs.

The Food and Drug Administration (FDA) has approved the following products:

- Selegiline
- Isocarboxzaid
- Phenelzine
- Tranylcypromine

Some of these medications are taken as pills, while others are applied to the skin as adhesive patches. Selegiline, for example, is available as a skin patch under the brand name Emsam.

What Is the Connection Between MAOIs, Tyramine, and the Diet?

Tyramine is a monoamine, which is a type of chemical compound. Dopamine, serotonin, and norepinephrine are examples of neurotransmitters.

According to a 2020 research, tyramine is a "trace" monoamine, which means that it is present in only trace amounts in animal tissues.

MAOIs can raise tyramine levels in the body. If someone taking an MAOI consumes foods high in tyramine, the levels of this chemical in the body can become dangerously high.

High tyramine levels can lead to:

- Headaches
- High blood pressure
- Brain Bleeds, if a person's blood pressure is extremely high.

Which Foods should a Person avoid?

Tyramine is not produced by the body, but eating and drinking foods and beverages high in tyramine will raise its level in the body.

Foods and beverages high in tyramine include:

- Cheese such as cheddar and feta cheeses
- Fermented vegetables such as Kimchi and sauerkraut
- Meats that have been cured or salt-dried
- Shrimp or fish that has been pickled or salt-dried
- Beer and wine
- Soy sauce
- Worcestershire sauce
- Chocolate.
- Coffee.
- Fresh fruits such as Avocado, grapes, and beets

Tyramine is also found in larger concentrations in older foods. As a result, anyone on MAOIs should avoid eating anything pickled, fermented, or overripe.

Precautions

a. MAOIs can interact with other medications.
b. Anyone using an MAOI should avoid taking a selective serotonin reuptake inhibitor (SSRI). When these two things are taken together, they can cause serotonin syndrome, which is when there is too much serotonin in the body.
c. MAOIs are the drugs that produce the most severe and prolonged episodes of serotonin syndrome.
d. Serotonin syndrome is potentially lethal. As a result, anyone taking an MAOI who has any of the following symptoms should seek medical attention immediately.
e. Serotonin syndrome symptoms include:
    - Restlessness and agitation
    - Anxiety
    - Disorientation
    - Vomiting and nausea
    - Perspiration
    - Rapid heartbeat
    - High body temperature
    - Muscle jerks and tremors
    - Muscle tightness
    - Hyperactive reflexes
    - Dilated pupils
    - Increased bowel sounds
    - Flushed skin
f. It is also risky to take more MAOI than advised or to combine this type of medication with another antidepressant.
g. Furthermore, anyone who has taken an MAOI within the last 10 days should avoid general anesthesia. This is done to avoid any

potentially harmful interactions between the antidepressant and the anesthesia.

What Are the Potential Negative Effects of MAOIs?

MAOIs can have a variety of adverse effects, the most prevalent of which are:

- Arid Mouth
- Nausea
- Diarrhea
- Constipation
- Drowsiness
- Insomnia
- Dizziness
- Lightheadedness

Furthermore, MAOI skin patches might occasionally induce skin responses.

Suicide and MAOIs

According to one 2018 study, antidepressant medications can raise the chance of suicidal thoughts, behavior, and death. These effects were most likely to be associated with SSRIs.

According to the study's authors, tricyclic antidepressants (TCAs) and noradrenergic and specific serotonergic antidepressants (NaSSAs) were only extremely rarely associated with these characteristics.

MAOIs were even less likely than TCAs and NaSSAs to be linked to suicide thoughts, actions, and death.

In summary

MAOIs are occasionally prescribed by doctors to treat depression, panic disorders, and social anxiety. The medications inhibit monoamine oxidase, an enzyme that degrades neurotransmitters in the brain.

But MAOIs have a lot of bad side effects, and doctors usually only use them as a last resort because there are other options.

To keep tyramine levels in the body from growing, those taking MAOIs should eat a limited diet. Also, never combine an MAOI and an SSRI, as this can result in serotonin syndrome, which can be fatal.

The Use Of Natural Supplements And Herbs In Treating Anxiety Disorders

Several herbal medicines have been studied as treatments for anxiety, but more research is needed to fully understand the risks and benefits. Here's what we know— and what we don't:

1. **Kava**: Kava appeared to be a potential anxiety treatment, but reports of substantial liver damage—even with short-term usage—prompted the Food and Drug Administration to publish warnings regarding the use of kava-containing dietary supplements. While the original reports of liver toxicity have been called into doubt, if you're thinking about using kava products, proceed with caution and consult with your doctor.

2. **Passion Flower**: A few tiny clinical investigations suggest that passion flower may aid with anxiety. Passion flower is often blended with other herbs in commercial products, making it difficult to differentiate the distinct properties of each herb. When taken as advised, passion flower is generally considered safe; however some studies have revealed that it can produce drowsiness, dizziness, and disorientation.

3. **Valerian**: People who consumed valerian reported less anxiety and tension in several studies. People in other research reported no advantage. Valerian is usually considered safe at recommended doses, but because long-term safety investigations are lacking, limit your use to a few weeks at a time unless your doctor allows. It may produce headaches, dizziness, and sleepiness as adverse effects.

4. **Chamomile**: Short-term usage of chamomile is generally deemed safe and can be useful in lowering anxiety symptoms, according to

limited studies. However, when used with blood-thinning medications, chamomile can increase the risk of bleeding. Some persons who are allergic to the plant family that contains chamomile may experience allergic responses if they use it. Ragweed, marigolds, daisies, and chrysanthemums are also members of this family.

5. Lavender: Some research suggests that taking lavender or using lavender aromatherapy helps alleviate anxiety; however, the evidence is preliminary and limited. Constipation and headaches might result from taking lavender orally. It can also stimulate appetite, make other drugs and supplements more sedative, and induce low blood pressure.

6. Lemon balm: According to preliminary study, lemon balm helps alleviate some anxiety symptoms such as anxiousness and excitability. Although lemon balm is generally well accepted and safe for short-term use, it might produce nausea and gastrointestinal pain.

The FDA does not regulate herbal supplements in the same way that medicines do. Despite improved quality control regulations in effect since 2010, the quality of some supplements may still be a concern. Remember that "natural" does not always imply "safe."

If you're thinking about using an herbal supplement to relieve anxiety, consult your doctor first, especially if you're taking other medications. Some herbal supplements can have major negative effects when combined with certain pharmaceuticals.

Some herbal remedies for anxiety can make you sleepy, making them unsafe to take while driving or performing dangerous duties. If you decide to try an herbal supplement, your doctor can help you understand the risks and advantages.

Consult your doctor if your anxiety is interfering with your everyday activities. For symptoms of more severe forms of anxiety to improve, medical treatment or psychological counseling (therapy) is usually required.

Understanding The Different Types Of Therapy For Treating Anxiety Disorders

All therapy approaches aim to help you understand why you feel the way you do, what your triggers are, and how you can change your response to them. Some types of therapy even teach you how to reframe negative thoughts and change your behavior.

Because anxiety disorders vary greatly, therapy is tailored to your specific symptoms and diagnosis. It can be done as an individual, family, couple, or group. The frequency and duration of your sessions with your therapist will be determined by your symptoms and diagnosis.

A. Cognitive-Behavioral Therapy

The most often used therapy for anxiety disorders is cognitive behavioral therapy (CBT). Studies have shown that it can help people with SAD, GAD, phobias, panic disorders, and other illnesses.

The assumption of CBT is that your ideas, not your current situation, influence how you feel and, as a result, how you behave. CBT's purpose is to discover and understand your negative thinking and inefficient behavior patterns and then replace them with more realistic beliefs, effective behaviors, and coping methods.

Throughout this process, your therapist serves as a coach, teaching you effective coping methods. For example, you may engage in a lot of "black-and-white" thinking, in which you presume that everything is either all evil or all good. Instead, you'd replace such thoughts with the more realistic experience of various shades of gray in between.

B. Exposure Therapy

Exposure therapy is a popular CBT technique for treating a wide range of anxiety disorders, including specific phobias, SAD, and PTSD. The core principle of exposure therapy is that facing your fears head-on is the best way to overcome them.

Your therapist will gradually expose you to anxiety-inducing things or situations during exposure therapy. This is often done with a method called "systematic desensitization," which has three steps:

Relax: To help you cope with your anxiety, your therapist will teach you relaxation techniques. Relaxation training includes things like progressive muscle relaxation, deep breathing, meditation, and guided imagery.

List: Make a list of your anxiety-inducing triggers and rate them in order of intensity.

Expose: In this last step, you'll slowly work through the things or situations that make you anxious, using relaxation techniques when you need to.

Your psychologist may subject you to anxiety-inducing stimuli in a variety of ways. The following are the most common:

Imaginal exposure: During this type of exposure, you will be told to think very clearly about the thing or situation that makes you anxious.

In this method, you will confront your anxiety-provoking object or situation in real life. As a result of this type of exposure, a person who suffers from social anxiety may be asked to give a speech in front of an audience.

Virtual reality exposure: When exposure in real life is not possible, virtual reality can be used. Virtual reality therapy uses technology to combine parts of exposure in real life and exposure in the mind. This strategy has been very beneficial for troops and those suffering from PTSD.

C. Dialectical Behavioral Therapy

Dialectical behavior therapy (DBT) is a kind of CBT that is extremely effective. DBT was developed to treat borderline personality disorder (BPD), but it is now used to treat a wide range of illnesses, including anxiety.

DBT emphasizes assisting you in developing what appears to be a "dialectical" (opposite) perspective, acceptance, and change. During DBT treatment, you will learn to accept your anxiety while also working hard to change it. It's comparable to the idea of accepting yourself as you are while still striving to improve yourself.

DBT therapy emphasizes four important skills:

Mindfulness: This is being able to focus on the present moment and watch fleeting thoughts, like anxiety, without letting them control you.

Stress tolerance: This is the ability to deal with your anxiety when something bad happens.

Interpersonal efficacy: This is the ability to say no or ask for what you require.

Emotion regulation: Managing anxiety before it becomes uncontrollable

D. Acceptance and Commitment Therapy

Acceptance and commitment therapy (ACT) is another type of therapy that has been shown to help with a variety of anxiety problems. ACT is about figuring out what your life values are and acting in ways that match those values.

ACT is made up of two major components:

- Accepting that thoughts and feelings do not have to be controlled.
- Making a commitment to do measures that will assist a person in living their life in accordance with their ideals.

ACT teaches people how to embrace their uncomfortable, nervous feelings. People don't try to get rid of their feelings or change them. Instead, they come up with ways to deal with them.

E. Art Therapy

Art therapy is a nonverbal, sensory-based therapy. It entails either expressing and processing emotion via visual art (painting, sketching, and sculpture) or practicing mindfulness and relaxation through art. Even though it can be used on its own, it is usually used along with other types of therapy, like CBT.

Since this is a newer type of therapy, more research needs to be done to show that it works to reduce anxiety symptoms.

F. Psychoanalytic Therapy

Anxiety symptoms, according to this Freudian concept, represent unconscious conflicts. The goal of psychoanalytic therapy is to help you resolve them. In psychoanalysis, you and your therapist look into your thoughts, fears, and desires to learn more about yourself and make you feel better. This is one of the most thorough forms of treatment; identifying patterns in your thinking might take years.

People sometimes use the terms "psychoanalysis" and "psychodynamic therapy" interchangeably. However, psychodynamic therapy is a type of psychoanalysis.

G. Interpersonal Therapy.

The focus of interpersonal therapy (IPT) is on social roles and relationships. During IPT, you and your therapist will look for any interpersonal problems you may be having, such as unresolved sadness, fights with family or friends, changes in your job or social roles, and problems with other people. Then, you'll learn how to talk about how you feel and how to communicate better with other people.

IPT was made to help people with severe depression, but it may also help people with SAD, whose anxiety is mostly caused by their relationships with other people.

Anxiety Therapy: What to Expect

A widespread misconception regarding treatment is that you will quickly feel better. This is not always the case. However, most of the time, you feel worse before you feel better. Surprisingly, feeling worse is frequently a sign of improvement. That makes sense when you think about it.

When you decide to go to therapy, it's usually because you haven't been able to work through your anxiety on your own. Therapy entails delving deeper and more meaningfully into your anxiety and its causes. This can temporarily increase your anxiety.

Therapy should never be considered a quick fix. It is a procedure that is unique to each person. The style of therapy you require, the skills you learn, and the length of time you spend in therapy are all determined by the type of anxiety you have and the severity of your symptoms.

It is critical to remember that, while the process will not always be pleasant, it will be entirely beneficial in the end.

Cognitive-Behavioral Therapy (CBT) and Its Effectiveness in Treating Anxiety Disorders

Cognitive-behavioral therapy (CBT) is a talking treatment that might help you manage your difficulties by altering your thinking and behavior.

It is widely used to treat anxiety and depression, but it can also help with other mental and physical health issues.

How CBT works in practice

CBT is founded on the idea that your thoughts, feelings, bodily sensations, and actions are all linked and that negative ideas and feelings can trap you in a downward spiral.

CBT helps you deal with problems that seem too big to handle in a more positive way by breaking them down into smaller parts.

You are told how to change these negative tendencies in order to feel better.

Unlike some other talking treatments, CBT focuses on current challenges rather than issues from the past.

It seeks practical strategies to improve your mental state on a daily basis.

CBT applications

CBT has been shown to help people with a wide range of mental health problems.

CBT can help people with, in addition to depression and anxiety disorders:

- Bipolar disorder.
- Borderline personality disorder.
- Eating disorders – such as anorexia and bulimia.
- Obsessive compulsive disorder (OCD).
- Panic attack.
- Phobias.
- Post-traumatic stress disorder (PTSD)
- Psychosis.
- Schizophrenia.
- Sleep problems – such as insomnia.
- Difficulties associated to alcohol consumption.

CBT is also used to treat people who have long-term health problems, such as:

- Irritable bowel syndrome (IBS).
- Chronic fatigue syndrome (CFS).
- Fibromyalgia.
- Chronic discomfort.

Although CBT cannot heal certain disorders' physical symptoms, it can help people cope with them better.

What Takes Place Throughout CBT Sessions

If CBT is indicated, you would normally meet with a therapist once a week or every two weeks.

Most treatments last between six and twenty sessions, and each session lasts between 30 and 60 minutes.

During the sessions, you and your therapist will work together to break down your problems into their component pieces, such as your ideas, physical feelings, and actions.

You and your therapist will examine these areas to see if they are unrealistic or harmful, and to see how they affect each other and you.

Then, your therapist will be able to help you figure out how to change unhelpful thoughts and actions.

After determining what you can alter, your therapist will ask you to put these adjustments into practice in your daily life, and you will discuss how you did during the next session.

The goal of therapy is to teach you how to use the skills you've learned in treatment in your everyday life.

This should help you deal with your problems and keep them from having a bad effect on your life even after your therapy is over.

Advantages and Disadvantages of Cognitive Behavioral Therapy (CBT)

Cognitive behavioral therapy (CBT) can help with some mental health problems, but it may not work or be the right choice for everyone.

CBT has several advantages, including:

- When compared to other talking therapies, it can be completed in a relatively short period of time.
- Because CBT is highly structured, it can be delivered in a variety of methods, including groups, self-help books, and online.

- It offers you helpful and practical tactics that you may use in your daily life even after the therapy is over.
- It emphasizes on the individual's ability to change (their thoughts, feelings and behaviors).
- It has the potential to be as successful as medicine in treating some mental health issues and may be useful in circumstances when medicine alone has failed.

The following downsides of CBT include:

- To get the most out of the procedure, you must commit to it; a therapist can assist and advise you, but they require your cooperation.
- Attending frequent CBT sessions and doing any extra work in between sessions might consume a significant amount of your time.
- It may not be appropriate for persons who have more significant mental health problems or learning disabilities.
- It entails confronting your emotions and fears - you may feel anxious or emotionally uncomfortable at first.
- It does not address any systemic or familial issues that may have a substantial impact on someone's health and well-being.

Some critics also say that CBT doesn't address the underlying causes of mental health problems, like a hard upbringing, even though it helps with present problems and focuses on specific problems.

Exposure Therapy And Its Effectiveness In Treating Anxiety Disorders

Exposure therapy is a type of therapy that helps people get over fears or worries that are caused by things, activities, or situations. Therapists and psychologists use it to treat conditions like post-traumatic stress disorder (PTSD) and phobias.

People tend to avoid things and situations that they are afraid of. According to the American Psychological Association, the idea behind exposure therapy is that exposing people to distressing stimuli in a safe setting helps them reduce avoidance and overcome their fear.

Therapists use exposure therapy to help people with phobias and anxiety get over them by breaking the cycle of fear and avoiding the things that make them scared. It works by exposing you to a fear-inducing stimulus in a safe atmosphere.

A person suffering from social anxiety, for example, may avoid going to crowded places like gatherings. A therapist would expose the person to these types of social settings during exposure therapy to help them become more comfortable in them.

Exposure treatment may be beneficial in four ways, according to experts:

Emotional processing: Exposure treatment aids in the development of realistic ideas about a frightening stimulus.

Extinction: Exposure therapy can help get rid of bad feelings about an object or situation that causes fear.

Habituation: Over time, repeated exposure to a frightening stimulus serves to reduce your reaction.

Self-efficacy: Exposure therapy shows you that you can get over your fears and deal with your anxiety.

Is There a Wide Range of Exposure Therapies?

According to the American Psychological Association, some potential exposure therapy variations include:

Vivo exposure: This entails confronting your fear in real life. Arachnophobics, for example, may interact with spiders.

Imaginal exposure: This occurs when a thing or situation is vividly imagined. A person who is afraid of birds, for example, might be asked to imagine themselves on a beach full of seagulls.

Exposure to virtual reality: Virtual reality technology can be used when it would be hard to face the source of fear in real life. A flight simulator, for example, could be used by someone who is afraid of flying.

Interoceptive exposure: This is a way to show that something is safe, even if it is feared, by causing a physical feeling. Someone who is afraid of lightheadedness because they believe it means they are having a stroke, for example, may be instructed to stand up quickly.

What diseases and conditions can exposure therapy help treat?

Exposure therapy is used to treat anxiety disorders such as the ones listed below:

- Generalized anxiety disorder.
- Obsessive-compulsive disorder (ocd).
- Phobias.
- Panic attack.
- Post-traumatic stress disorder.
- Social anxiety disorder.

How Can I Find An Exposure Treatment Specialist

Exposure therapy is a sort of cognitive-behavioral treatment that is usually administered by a therapist, psychologist, or psychiatrist.

Here are some pointers to consider while selecting a specialist:

- Start your search with sites you can trust, such as the American Psychological Association's website.
- Check with a national organization or network that specializes in your disease, such as the National Center for PTSD.
- Look for feedback from those who have worked with the specialist.
- Inquire with someone you trust about a mental health doctor they've worked with. You can also seek referrals from your primary care provider.

Ask questions such as:

- How much experience you have working with [your issue].
- What is your area of specialization?
- What can we do if exposure therapy fails?

If you're paying via insurance, check your provider's directory or see if they cover out-of-network therapists in circumstances where exposure treatment isn't covered by your plan.

Can I Subject Myself To Exposure Therapy

Most of the time, exposure therapy is done with the help of a therapist or another medical professional. A small review of research published in 2018 showed that therapist-led exposure therapy was more effective at treating OCD symptoms than self-led treatment.

If you try exposure therapy without the help of a trained professional, you might end up with more stress or fear. You should not attempt to cure a serious disorder like PTSD on your own.

You could use parts of exposure therapy in your everyday life to help you get over mild phobias.

It's a natural human propensity to avoid things and situations that make you uncomfortable. Forcing yourself to confront your fears may assist you in stepping outside of your comfort zone.

For example, if you have mild social anxiety, you might feel nervous when you're in a crowd or at a get-together. You can try to compel yourself to spend more time in increasingly crowded settings.

In summary

Therapists employ exposure therapy to help you overcome your fear. Exposition therapy has been shown in studies to be useful in treating a number of anxiety disorders, including PTSD and phobias.

Exposure treatment should be done under the direction of a skilled specialist. The American Psychological Association website is one place to look for specialists in your area.

Acceptance And Commitment Therapy (ACT) And Its Effectiveness In Treating Anxiety Disorders

Acceptance and commitment therapy (ACT) is a type of psychotherapy that focuses on accepting negative thoughts, feelings, symptoms, or situations. It also makes you more likely to stick with healthy, positive activities that help you reach your goals or ideals.

Therapists who use ACT follow a philosophy that says more acceptance can make people more adaptable. This method has a number of benefits, and it may help people break the habit of avoiding certain thoughts or feelings, which can lead to problems later on.

Unlike CBT, the goal of ACT is not to reduce the frequency or intensity of unpleasant internal experiences like upsetting cognitive distortions, emotions, or drives. Instead, the goal is to make it easier for you to control or get rid of unwanted feelings while making it easier for you to take part in important life activities that are in line with your personal values.

This procedure consists of six steps:

A. **Acceptance:** This means letting your own thoughts and feelings come up without trying to change them or ignore them. Acceptance is a dynamic process.

B. **Cognitive defusion**: This is the process of distancing yourself from your inner experiences. This lets you see your thoughts as they are without attaching any importance to them.

C. **Self as context**: This entails learning to separate your views about yourself from your actions.

D. **Being present**: ACT helps you to be aware of your surroundings and to learn to shift your focus away from internal thoughts and feelings.

E. **Values**: These are the aspects of your life that are significant enough to encourage you to take action.

F. **Commitment**: This phase entails adjusting your behavior in accordance with the principles discussed in treatment.

During ACT, your therapist will teach you how to use these concepts in your daily life. They may help you learn how to practice acceptance and cognitive defusion, or they may help you get a sense of yourself that is separate from your emotions and feelings.

Mindfulness exercises may also be used in sessions. These are meant to help people become more aware of thoughts, feelings, sensations, and memories that they have been avoiding. Your therapist may also be able to help you figure out when your actions don't match up with what you believe and what actions might.

Your therapist may offer you homework, such as mindfulness, cognitive, or value-clarifying activities, to do between sessions. You and your therapist decide what your homework will be, and it can be changed to be as helpful and personal as possible.

What Can ACT Do For You

Anxiety and depression may benefit from ACT therapy. Other benefits of ACT therapy include:

- Eating disorders
- Obsessive-compulsive disorder (OCD)
- Stress
- Substance use
- Psychosis

ACT has been shown in studies to improve symptoms in people with generalized anxiety disorder (GAD), and it may be an especially good fit for older adults with the condition.

The Advantages of ACT

One of the most important advantages of ACT is the effect it has on psychological flexibility. Psychological flexibility is being able to accept and let go of your thoughts and feelings when it makes sense to do so. This allows you to respond intelligently to your inner experience and avoid short-term, impulsive acts, instead concentrating on living a meaningful life.

Being mentally flexible can help you deal with the symptoms of disorders like anxiety and depression. Because of this increase in mental flexibility, these symptoms may often get much better in a big way.

ACT's Effectiveness

ACT is sometimes known as "third wave" or "new wave" psychotherapy. The term "third wave" treatment applies to a wide range of psychotherapies, including:

- Behavioral Dialectical Therapy (DBT).
- Schema therapy.
- Mindfulness-Based Cognitive Therapy (MBCT).

In the past, it was thought that third-wave treatments were best for people who had not gotten better from other treatments, like traditional CBT. However, it is currently thought that for some people, third-wave therapy may make sense as a first-line treatment.

According to research, ACT is useful in treating a wide range of diseases, including those that transcend multiple diagnoses. ACT also seems to improve the quality of life and may help with physical problems and long-term pain.

What to Consider

Even though ACT is a good way to treat a number of disorders, research suggests that it may be about as effective as other therapies, like CBT.

These results suggest that a person who does well with ACT may also do well with another treatment.

ACT has also been chastised for being too similar to other types of therapy. Some CBT supporters argue that ACT, like other third-wave therapies, does not take a significantly different approach.

Getting Started

ACT can be given by psychiatrists, psychologists, social workers, mental health counselors, and others who work in mental health. If you want to learn more about this method, you can ask your therapist if they have been trained in it or look for an ACT practitioner with a lot of experience.

You could also contact the Association for Contextual Behavioral Science (ACBS) or the Association for Behavioral and Cognitive Therapies (ABCT). The ACBS also gives away free ACT tools like films, audio clips, and activities that help you be more aware.

During the sessions, an ACT-trained therapist will be both an active, empathic listener and an active guide, encouraging deeper investigation and nonjudgmental awareness.

ACT sessions are typically interactive, with psychological exercises or mindfulness training as well as homework assigned following the session. Doing these activities is an important part of ACT because it helps you learn new skills and makes you more mentally flexible.

During therapy, your therapist will also want to address your beliefs and ambitions. This is an important part of your treatment because these values will guide what you do in the future.

Family Therapy and Its Effectiveness in Treating Anxiety Disorders

What is Family Therapy?

The term "family therapy" suggests that family members seek psychotherapy as a group.

Though it is beneficial if everyone in the family participates, family therapy does not require your entire family to be involved.

This means that the therapy will concentrate on family connections and dynamics.

Family counseling is often brief and focused on specific goals. It investigates the patterns, tensions, and communication styles in your family system.

Family counseling may benefit you and your family in the following ways:

- Increasing communication abilities.
- Offering tools for coping with hard situations.
- Bringing new insight and comprehension.
- Recognizing issue areas within the household.
- Giving ideas for handling conflict.

Relationships are being improved and strengthened.

Family therapy may be led by one of the evidence-based treatment approaches listed below, or your therapist may combine aspects of many approaches.

Approaches To Family Therapy

Let's look more closely at the most common approaches used in family therapy:

A. Systemic family therapy

This therapy method views the family as a unit in which each member's activities affect the other members and the family as a whole.

Therapy aims to improve family interactions by better understanding family dynamics, how they affect people, and how they develop over time.

B. Structural family therapy

Salvador Minuchin created structural family therapy in the 1960s. It is based on the idea that emotional and behavioral problems in children and teens are often caused by broken family structures.

Treatment focuses on helping people understand the boundaries and subsystems of their families so that everyone can work together better.

It also focuses on establishing proper limits and building family relationships.

C. Brief strategic family therapy.

This method of therapy is often restricted to 12 sessions. The goal is to find and change the ways in which a child, teen, or young adult interacts with their family that contribute to their bad behavior.

Most likely, the therapist will work to reinforce good habits and change bad family habits that hurt a young child in crisis.

The therapist will probably also give the family tasks to look at and improve how they talk to each other.

D. Psycho-education

Family therapy often includes opportunities to learn about mental health problems that affect family relationships as well as treatments that have been shown to work.

One tiny study published in 2018 found that educating a family enhances the way the entire family functions.

A 2006 study found that people with mental health conditions have a better outlook and have fewer relapses when their families understand their conditions better and are better able to help each other.

What should you anticipate from a family therapy session?

Certain goals are frequently shared by family therapies. Typically, these are:

- Investigating how family members interact with one another
- Detecting and improving any harmful communication practices in the family system.
- Marshaling the family's strengths and resources.

- Providing the family with improved problem-solving abilities.

Even though each therapist has their own way of doing things, here is a general idea of what family therapy may involve:

The Initial Steps

During your first meeting with your therapist, you and your family will probably talk about the problem that brought you and your family to therapy.

Your therapist will give each participant the opportunity to discuss what they believe are the most important issues that they or their family is dealing with and why.

Assessment

During the next several sessions, your therapist will most likely gather information from you in order to develop a picture of your family and how it functions, including:

- Your family history.
- Family roles.
- Parenting and disciplinary techniques.
- Coping skills your family has utilized.

Your therapist will gain a grasp of your family's difficulties and how you responded to them collectively and individually.

Your therapist may urge you to consider and write about who in your family has power and how decisions are made.

If your therapist approaches family therapy strategically, you may address how the problem that brought you to treatment serves a specific function in your family.

If your family used certain ways to cope, you may be asked to think about and talk about whether or not those ways are still helpful.

Mapping the Family Structure

If your therapist uses a structural approach, the next step might be for him or her to make a map of your family that shows the order of power.

The map might help you explain how power and limits work in your family, especially how they might change over time.

Developing A Therapeutic Strategy

Family therapists are often more engaged in finding solutions to problems than in assigning blame.

Working together, you and your therapist will most likely develop a plan outlining what you and any family members who are participating in treatment can do to improve problematic communication and problem-solving behaviors.

Your therapy plan may also include strategies for enhancing your family's unique strengths.

Family Therapist Education And Training

Most of the time, a mental health professional who has had formal training in psychotherapy for couples or family systems is the one who does family therapy.

Most family therapists have master's or PhD degrees in a field of mental health that focuses on marriage and family therapy.

To become state-licensed, marriage and family therapists must complete a supervised clinical fellowship (usually two years).

The Association of Marital and Family Therapy Regulatory Boards also requires therapists with a master's degree to pass a test.

On the other hand, the exam for therapists with PhDs is run by the Association of State and Provincial Psychology Boards.

How to Choose the Best Therapist for Your Family

It is critical for the effectiveness of your therapy to find the right therapist for you and your family. To locate a good fit, it's fine to take your time, ask questions, check credentials, and even "interview" therapists.

Here are some things to think about:

- Is the therapist in your state licensed?
- Is the therapist familiar with assisting families dealing with similar issues?
- In treatment, do you feel heard and supported?
- Is this therapist in your network if you have health insurance?
- How close is the therapist's office to your house or workplace?
- Is the therapist able to provide virtual mental health services?

The American Association for Marriage and Family Therapy may be able to help you identify a marriage and family therapist.

In summary

Family therapy is a type of psychotherapy that focuses on family dynamics and the development of more positive interactions within family systems. It can be especially beneficial if you or a member of your family suffers from:

- Interpersonal or financial troubles.
- Marital issues.
- Problem with substance misuse.
- Mental health condition.

With the help of your therapist, you and your family members can look at your family's problem-solving skills, boundaries, systems of authority, and ways of communicating to find patterns that could be troublesome.

Then, your therapist will work with you to make a plan for improving how your family communicates and solves problems.

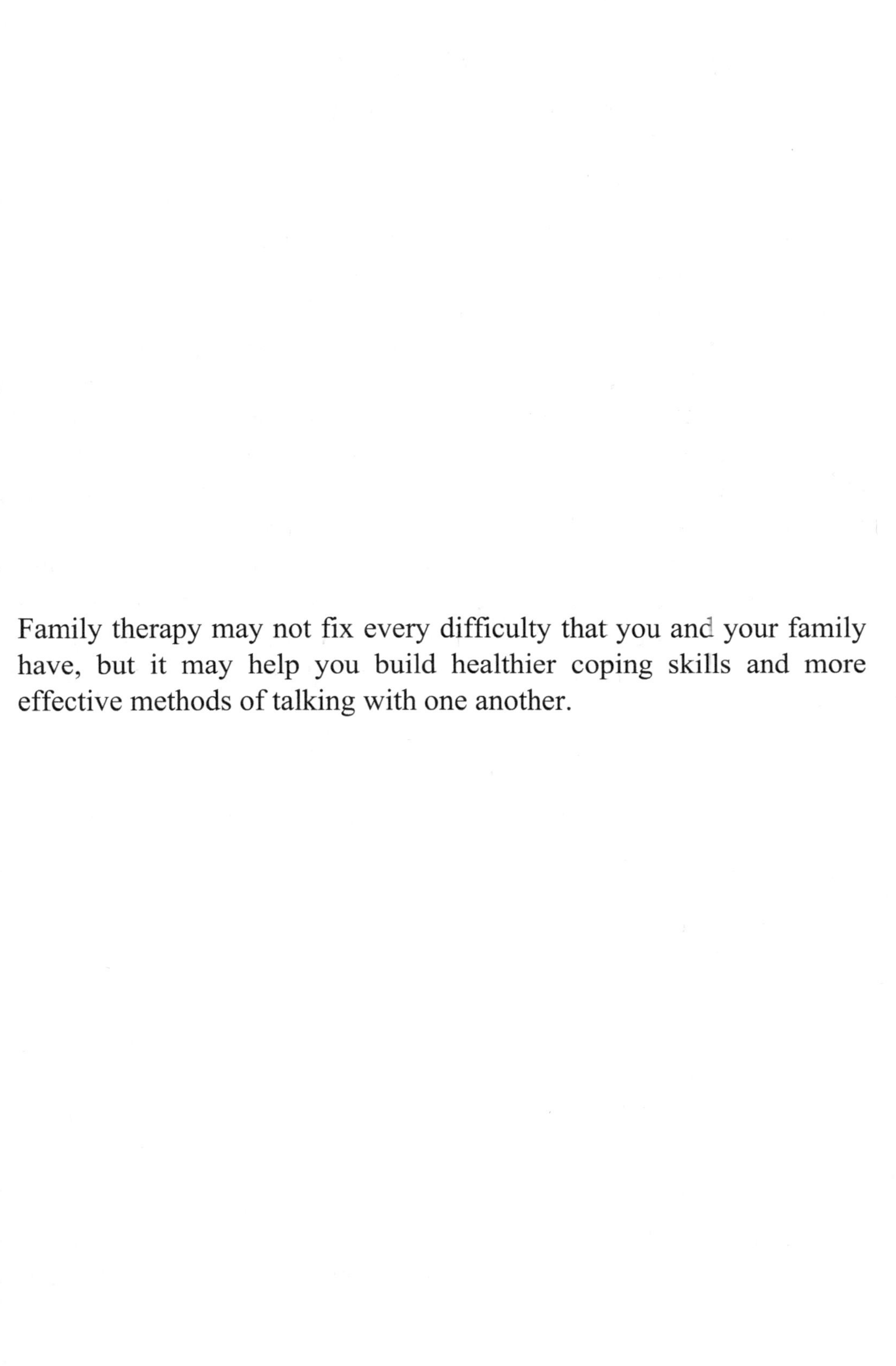

Family therapy may not fix every difficulty that you and your family have, but it may help you build healthier coping skills and more effective methods of talking with one another.

COPING STRATEGIES FOR SPECIFIC ANXIETY DISORDERS

"Coping strategies" are the different ways that people with anxiety disorders can deal with their symptoms in a healthy way. Different anxiety disorders have different symptoms and levels of severity, so they need different ways to be treated. Some common anxiety disorders include Generalized Anxiety Disorder (GAD), Panic Disorder, Social Anxiety Disorder, Specific Phobias, and Obsessive-Compulsive Disorder. Effective ways to deal with these disorders could involve a mix of therapy, medication, self-care techniques, and changes to the way you live. It is important for people to work with their mental health professional to come up with a plan to deal with their symptoms and needs that is unique to them. Also, coping methods may need to be changed over time as symptoms change and as new problems come up. The main goal of coping strategies is to reduce anxiety, make it easier to get through the day, and improve overall health.

Coping Strategies For Panic Disorder

A panic attack is a sudden and acute feeling of anxiety.

Physical signs of panic episodes can include:

- shaking
- Feelings of disorientation
- Nausea
- Fast and irregular Heartbeats
- Arid mouth
- breathlessness
- sweating
- dizziness

A panic attack's symptoms are not hazardous, although they can be scary. They can make you feel as if you're having a heart attack, about to collapse, or even about to die. The majority of panic attacks last between 5 and 30 minutes.

How To Deal With A Panic Attack

It is critical not to allow your fear of panic attacks to control you.

Panic attacks always pass, and the symptoms are not indicative of anything dangerous. Tell yourself that the symptoms you're having are the result of anxiety.

Avoid looking for diversions. Survive the assault. Continue to do your best. If at all feasible, attempt to stay in the scenario until the worry subsides.

Face your fears. If you don't run away from it, you're giving yourself the opportunity to learn that nothing will happen.

As the worry goes away, pay attention to your surroundings again and do what you were doing before.

If you're having a short, unexpected panic attack, having someone with you can help reassure you that it will pass and the symptoms are nothing to worry about.

Breathing Practice To Help With Panic Attacks

If you're having a panic attack and are breathing quickly, completing a breathing exercise will help relieve your other symptoms. Consider this:

- Breathe in through your nostrils as slowly, deeply, and gently as you can.
- Through your mouth, exhale slowly, deeply, and gently.
- Some people find it beneficial to count from 1 to 5 on each in-breath and out-breath.
- Focus on your breathing and close your eyes.
- Within a few minutes, you should begin to feel better. You can feel exhausted afterwards.

Methods For Avoiding Panic Attacks

- You should try to figure out what specific stressors are causing your symptoms to worsen. It is critical not to limit your regular activities and movements.
- Do breathing exercises every day to help prevent panic attacks and to help relieve them when they occur.
- Regular exercise, especially aerobic exercise, can help you deal with stress, release tension, improve your mood, and boost your confidence.
- Consume regular meals to keep your blood sugar levels stable.
- Avoid coffee, alcohol, and smoking, as these might aggravate panic episodes.
- To gain valuable advice on how to manage your panic attacks, try a panic support group - your GPS can put you in contact with groups in your area.

To identify and change the negative thought patterns that are fueling your panic episodes, try cognitive behavioral therapy (CBT).

Is it a panic attack?

If you are always upset and worried, especially about when your next panic attack will happen, you may have panic disorder.

People suffering from panic disorder may avoid circumstances that could trigger an attack. They may also be afraid of and avoid public places (agoraphobia).

There is no quick treatment, but if your attacks continue, seek medical attention.

Coping Strategies For Phobias

Phobias are intense and irrational fears of specific objects or situations, such as heights, enclosed spaces, or animals. Coping strategies for phobias include both therapy and self-help techniques.

- **Cognitive-behavioral therapy (CBT):** This type of therapy focuses on changing negative thought patterns and behaviors associated with phobias. Techniques such as exposure therapy, in which a person is gradually exposed to their phobia in a controlled setting, can help to reduce the fear response.
- **Mindfulness and relaxation techniques:** Being mindful and taking deep breaths can help reduce anxiety in the moment, while progressive muscle relaxation and guided imagery can help reduce stress and tension.
- **Challenge negative thoughts**: Identifying and challenging negative beliefs associated with the phobia can help to reduce fear and anxiety.
- **Seek support**: Talking to friends and family or joining a support group can provide a sense of community and help reduce feelings of isolation and anxiety.
- **Gradual exposure**: Gradually exposing oneself to the object or situation they fear can help reduce the anxiety response. It is important to start with small, manageable steps and work up to larger exposures.
- **Medication**: In severe cases, medication may be prescribed to help reduce symptoms of anxiety and phobia.

It is important to remember that everyone's experience with phobias is different, and what works for one person may not work for another. To deal with phobia symptoms, it's important to work with a mental health professional to make a plan that fits your needs.

Coping Strategies For Social Anxiety Disorder (SAD)

Social anxiety disorder is a type of anxiety disorder that causes a lot of fear and embarrassment around other people. It can be difficult for people with social anxiety disorder to interact with others, attend events, or perform in front of others. However, there are coping strategies that can help manage the symptoms of social anxiety disorder and improve one's quality of life.

- **Gradual exposure**: Gradual exposure to feared social situations can help people with social anxiety disorder overcome their fears. This can be done by starting with small, less threatening situations and gradually working up to more challenging situations.
- **Mindfulness and relaxation techniques**: Mindfulness and relaxation techniques, such as deep breathing and progressive muscle relaxation, can help reduce anxiety in social situations.
- **Cognitive-behavioral therapy (CBT)**: CBT is a form of therapy that focuses on changing negative thought patterns and behaviors. CBT can help people with social anxiety disorder question and change their negative thoughts about being in social situations.
- **Medications:** Anti-anxiety medications, such as selective serotonin reuptake inhibitors (SSRIs), can help reduce symptoms of social anxiety disorder.
- **Support groups**: Joining a support group of people with similar experiences can provide a sense of community and reduce feelings of isolation.
- **Practice social skills**: Practicing social skills in a safe and controlled environment, such as role-playing exercises, can help build confidence and reduce anxiety in social situations.
- **Seek professional help**: A mental health professional can help develop a treatment plan tailored to the individual's specific needs and provide guidance and support throughout the process.

It is important to remember that everyone is different, and what works for one person may not work for another. To deal with social anxiety disorder, it's important to work with a mental health professional to make a personalized plan and find the best ways to cope.

Coping Strategies For Generalized Anxiety Disorder

Generalized Anxiety Disorder (GAD) is a mental health condition characterized by persistent, excessive, and unrealistic worry about various aspects of life, such as health, work, money, or relationships. The anxiety is not focused on a specific event or situation and can be difficult to control. Coping strategies for GAD can include a combination of self-help techniques, therapy, and medication.

- **Mindfulness techniques**: Mindfulness practices, such as meditation and deep breathing, can help individuals with GAD become more aware of their thoughts and feelings and reduce their worry.
- **Cognitive-behavioral therapy (CBT):** CBT can help people with GAD learn to recognize and question negative thoughts and beliefs that make them anxious.
- **Exercise:** Regular physical activity can help to reduce symptoms of anxiety and improve overall well-being.
- **Relaxation techniques**: Relaxation techniques, such as progressive muscle relaxation, can help to reduce physical tension and calm the mind.
- **Sleep hygiene**: Good sleep hygiene can help individuals with GAD get a good night's sleep, which can reduce symptoms of anxiety and improve overall mood.
- **Medication:** Antidepressants, beta-blockers, and benzodiazepines are among the medications that can be used to treat GAD. Medication should always be prescribed and monitored by a mental health professional.
- **Lifestyle changes**: Making changes to diet and exercise can help reduce symptoms of GAD. Limiting caffeine and alcohol can also help reduce symptoms.
- **Social support**: Building a strong support system of friends and family can help individuals with GAD feel less isolated and more empowered to manage their condition.

It is important to remember that everyone with GAD is different, and the coping strategies that work best for one person may not work as well for another. Some people may need to use a mix of ways to deal with their GAD in order to handle it well.

Mindfulness And Relaxation Techniques For Managing Panic Disorder

Panic disorder is a type of anxiety disorder that is marked by repeated panic attacks. Panic attacks are sudden, intense bouts of fear that can be accompanied by physical symptoms like palpitations, sweating, shaking, shortness of breath, and chest pain. The fear of having another panic attack can also cause a lot of stress and make it hard to get through the day.

Mindfulness and relaxation techniques can help people with panic disorder deal with their symptoms by making them feel less stressed and more calm. With these techniques, you focus on the present moment and become more aware of your thoughts, feelings, and bodily sensations.

Here are some examples of mindfulness and relaxation techniques that can help people with panic disorder:

- **Deep breathing exercises**: This involves taking slow, deep breaths and focusing on the sensation of air entering and leaving the body.
- **Progressive muscle relaxation**: This technique involves tensing and relaxing muscle groups to release physical tension and reduce stress.
- **Guided imagery and visualization**: This involves using your imagination to visualize calming scenes or scenarios.
- **Mindful movement**: This involves engaging in physical activities such as yoga, tai chi, or qigong, which involve moving slowly and mindfully to reduce stress and increase relaxation.

- **Mindfulness-based stress reduction (MBSR)**: This involves using mindfulness techniques to reduce stress and improve overall well-being.

By using these techniques every day, you can help deal with panic disorder and feel less anxious. It's important to remember that these techniques work best when combined with other evidence-based treatments such as cognitive-behavioral therapy (CBT) and medication.

Exposure Therapy For Phobias: Understanding The Process And How To Use It

Exposure therapy is a type of cognitive-behavioral therapy that aims to reduce anxiety and fear in response to specific stimuli, such as phobias. It works by slowly exposing the person to the thing, situation, or experience they are afraid of in a safe, controlled setting. This type of therapy is based on the idea that confronting a feared stimulus can help to decrease anxiety and improve the person's overall quality of life.

Exposure therapy starts with an assessment of the phobia and the creation of a hierarchy of feared stimuli. The person is then gradually exposed to the feared stimuli, starting with the least feared and working up to the most feared. The therapist helps the person face the stimuli in a safe, controlled, and supportive environment and helps the person manage their anxiety while they are exposed to the stimuli. To help the person get over their fear, the therapist may use relaxation techniques, cognitive restructuring, and other ways to deal with stress.

Exposure therapy can be effective for phobias as well as for other anxiety disorders such as panic disorder, social anxiety disorder, and obsessive-compulsive disorder. It can take time to see results, but exposure therapy is considered to be one of the most effective treatments for phobias and other anxiety disorders. It's important to remember that exposure therapy should only be done by someone who has been trained to do it.

Cognitive-Behavioral Therapy (CBT) For Social Anxiety Disorder: Understanding The Process And How To Use It

Cognitive-behavioral therapy (CBT) is a common and effective way to treat social anxiety disorder (SAD). It is based on the idea that the way we think about ourselves, the world, and other people affects the way we feel and behave.

CBT for SAD typically involves the following steps:

- **Education**: The therapist will educate the patient about SAD and its causes, including the role of negative thoughts and beliefs.
- **Identifying negative thoughts**: The therapist will help the patient identify negative thoughts and beliefs that contribute to their social anxiety.
- **Challenging negative thoughts**: The therapist will help the patient challenge and replace these negative thoughts with more realistic and positive ones.
- **In vivo exposure:** The patient will go through exposure therapy, in which they gradually face their fears in a controlled setting.
- **Behavior change**: The therapist will help the patient change their behavior in social situations by practicing new coping skills and challenging their negative thoughts.
- **Maintenance**: The therapist will work with the patient to develop a plan for maintaining their progress and preventing relapse.
- **Homework**: The patient may be given homework assignments to reinforce what they have learned in therapy and to practice their new coping skills outside of therapy sessions.

Patients with SAD can use CBT to learn how to recognize and question their negative thoughts and beliefs, gain more confidence in social situations, and learn new ways to deal with their anxiety. With time and practice, they can get a better view of themselves, feel less anxious, and live a better life.

Medications For Generalized Anxiety Disorder: Understanding The Different Types Of Medications And How They Work

Generalized anxiety disorder (GAD) is a common mental health problem that causes people to worry and be afraid all the time. There are several medications that can be used to treat GAD, including:

- **Antidepressants**: Selective serotonin reuptake inhibitors (SSRIs) and serotonin-norepinephrine reuptake inhibitors (SNRIs) are commonly prescribed for GAD. These medications help to balance chemicals in the brain and can reduce symptoms such as worry, fear, and insomnia. Examples include fluoxetine, escitalopram, and venlafaxine.
- **Benzodiazepines**: These medications are sometimes used to treat symptoms of anxiety, including panic attacks and insomnia. They work quickly but can be habit-forming and should be used only for short-term treatment. Examples include lorazepam and alprazolam.
- **Beta-blockers:** These drugs are mostly used to treat problems with the heart, but they can also help ease anxiety symptoms like a fast heartbeat and sweating. They are not usually used as a first-line treatment for GAD.

It's important to note that these medications are not a cure for GAD, but they can help relieve symptoms so that individuals can participate in therapy or other treatments. Additionally, medication may not be appropriate for everyone, and side effects can occur. It's best to discuss the risks and benefits of these medications with a healthcare provider.

Coping With Physical Symptoms Of Anxiety Disorders

Coping with the physical symptoms of anxiety disorders can be challenging, but there are some strategies that may help. Here are a few ways to manage physical symptoms:

- **Relaxation techniques**: Practicing deep breathing, progressive muscle relaxation, and yoga can help reduce physical symptoms of anxiety.
- **Exercise**: Regular physical activity can help reduce muscle tension and improve sleep, which can alleviate physical symptoms of anxiety.
- **Mindfulness**: Mindfulness techniques can help you focus on the present moment and avoid getting caught up in anxiety-provoking thoughts and feelings.
- **Cognitive restructuring**: Challenging and reframing negative thoughts and beliefs can help reduce physical symptoms of anxiety.
- **Medications**: Antidepressant and antianxiety medications can help regulate heart rate and breathing, as well as reducing muscle tension and fatigue.
- **Therapy**: Talking with a therapist can help you understand and manage physical symptoms of anxiety and develop coping skills.

If physical symptoms of anxiety are getting in the way of your daily life, you should see a doctor. A health care professional can help you figure out what the best way is to treat your symptoms.

Support Groups and Self-Help Resources for Coping With Anxiety Disorders

People with anxiety disorders can get a lot of help and information from support groups and self-help materials. These resources can include:

- **Online forums and support groups**: Many online forums and support groups offer a safe and supportive space to connect with others who have similar experiences with anxiety.
- **Books and self-help materials**: There are many books and self-help materials available on anxiety disorders, including information on coping strategies and treatments.

- **Professional therapy and counseling**: Professional therapy and counseling can provide individuals with the opportunity to work one-on-one with a mental health professional to develop coping strategies and manage their anxiety.
- **Medication management**: Medications can be a helpful tool in managing symptoms of anxiety disorders, and individuals can work with a healthcare provider to develop a medication plan.
- **Mind-body practices such as mindfulness meditation and yoga**: These practices can help individuals to manage anxiety symptoms by reducing stress and promoting relaxation.

It is important for individuals to find the resources and coping strategies that work best for them, as everyone's experience with anxiety is unique.

BUILDING RESILIENCE AND DEVELOPING A SUPPORT NETWORK

Building resilience and developing a support network are crucial components of managing anxiety disorders. Resilience is a person's ability to deal with stress and hard times and to get back on their feet after a setback. A strong support network includes friends, family, and healthcare professionals who can offer emotional support, encouragement, and practical help.

A strong support network can give people a sense of belonging, lessen feelings of loneliness and isolation, and help them come up with healthy ways to deal with problems. To build resilience, people need to learn skills and form habits that help them deal with stress in a more positive and helpful way. This could mean taking care of yourself, having a positive attitude, being physically active, and getting professional help when you need it.

Mindfulness and relaxation techniques can also help you build up your ability to deal with stress and anxiety. Mindfulness means being in the present, paying attention to your thoughts and feelings, and letting them be as they are without judging them. Deep breathing, progressive muscle relaxation, and guided imagery are all examples of relaxation techniques that can help people deal with the physical symptoms of anxiety and feel less stressed and tense.

In the end, building resilience and making a network of support are important ways to deal with anxiety and improve overall health. By using these strategies every day, people can build a more positive and resilient attitude and take charge of their mental health.

Understanding Resilience And How To Build It

Resilience is the capacity to bounce back from adversity, trauma, or stress. It refers to the ability of individuals to adapt to and recover from difficult experiences and maintain their well-being. Resilience is a key part of keeping your mental health in good shape, and it is essential for dealing with stress and anxiety. Understanding what resilience is and how to build it can have a big effect on a person's quality of life as a whole.

There are several key factors that contribute to resilience, including having strong social support networks, developing a positive outlook and healthy coping mechanisms, and maintaining a healthy lifestyle. Building resilience can take time and effort, but there are many practical strategies that individuals can use to strengthen their resilience and better cope with life's challenges.

One of the best ways to build resilience is to do regular physical activities, like yoga or exercise, and eat a healthy diet that gives the body the nutrients it needs. Engaging in mindfulness practices, such as meditation or journaling, can also help to build resilience by reducing stress levels and promoting positive thinking.

Having a positive outlook and doing things that bring you joy and satisfaction is also important for building resilience. This might include volunteering, pursuing hobbies, or simply spending time with loved ones. Seeking help from friends, family, or support groups is also important for building resilience, because having a strong social network can make people feel safe and secure.

In conclusion, understanding resilience and how to build it is an important part of managing anxiety and stress. People can better deal with life's challenges and keep their mental health if they take steps to build resilience and do things that promote well-being.

Coping With Stress: How To Manage Stress In A Healthy Way

Managing stress in a healthy way can be an important aspect of fighting against anxiety disorder. Here are some ways to manage stress in a healthy manner:

A. **Exercise regularly**: Physical activity such as jogging, yoga, or even a simple walk can help release tension, improve mood, and reduce stress levels.

B. **Practice mindfulness and meditation**: Mindfulness practices such as deep breathing, meditation, and yoga can help calm the mind and reduce stress.

C. **Connect with others**: Spending time with friends, family, or a support group can provide emotional support and help reduce feelings of isolation and loneliness.

D. **Get enough sleep**: Aim for 7-9 hours of sleep per night to help improve mood, focus, and reduce stress levels.

E. **Healthy eating**: Eating a balanced diet that includes plenty of fruits, vegetables, whole grains, and lean protein can provide the body with the necessary nutrients to help manage stress.

F. **Limit caffeine and alcohol**: Caffeine and alcohol can interfere with sleep patterns, increase anxiety and disrupt mood, so it's important to limit their consumption.

G. **Try relaxation techniques.** Relaxation techniques like progressive muscle relaxation, visualizing, or aromatherapy can help reduce tension and help you feel more relaxed.

H. **Get involved in activities you enjoy**: Engaging in activities you enjoy, such as reading, listening to music, or painting, can help distract you from stress and provide a healthy outlet for emotions.

By implementing these healthy stress management techniques, it can help individuals better manage anxiety disorders and reduce the negative impact stress can have on their lives.

10 Practical Ways to Manage Stress

It's difficult not to feel overwhelmed now and then. You can become overly stressed and occupied juggling work, family, and other commitments. However, you must make time to relax, or your mental and physical health may suffer.

It takes practice to learn how to regulate your stress, but you can and must do it. Here are ten suggestions to help:

A. Exercise.

Working out on a daily basis is one of the most effective ways to calm your body and mind. Exercise will also boost your mood. However, you must do it frequently for it to be effective.

So, how much exercise should you do each week?

Work up to 2 hours and 30 minutes of moderately intense exercise, such as brisk walks, or 75 minutes of rigorous exercise, such as swimming laps, jogging, or participating in sports.

Set exercise objectives that you can achieve so that you don't give up. Most importantly, remember that any activity is preferable to none at all.

B. Stretch Your Muscles

Your muscles tense up when you're stressed. You may help loosen them up and refresh your body on your own by:

- Exercising.
- Relaxing with a massage.
- Enjoying a warm bath or shower.
- Having a restful night's sleep.

C. Deep Inhalation.

Stopping and taking a few deep breaths can immediately relieve stress. You'll be astonished at how much better you'll feel once you've mastered it. Simply follow these 5 steps:

- Sit in a comfortable position, hands on your lap, feet on the floor. You can also lie down.
- Shut your eyes.
- Visualize yourself in a relaxing environment. It may be on the beach, in a magnificent field of grass, or someplace else that makes you feel serene.
- Take slow, deep breaths in and out.
- Repeat for 5–10 minutes at a time.

D. Eat Healthily

Eating a well-balanced meal on a daily basis will help you feel better in general. It may also aid in mood regulation. For energy, your meals should be high in vegetables, fruit, whole grains, and lean protein.

E. Be patient

Modern life is so hectic that sometimes we just need to sit down and relax. Look around your life for simple ways to do this. The following are examples:

- Set your watch to 5 to 10 minutes ahead of time. You'll arrive a little earlier and escape the worry of being late.
- Switch to the slow lane when driving on the highway to avoid road rage.
- Divide large tasks into smaller ones. For example, if you don't have to, don't try to answer all 100 emails; instead, respond to a handful of them.

F. Take a breather.

You should schedule some genuine downtime to give your mind a break from stress. If you like to establish objectives, this may be difficult for you at first. But if you stay with it, you'll start looking forward to these moments. You can relax by doing the following:

- Meditation
- Yoga
- Tai chi
- Prayer
- Playing your favorite music
- Spending time outside in nature

G. Set aside time for hobbies.

You must make time for activities that you enjoy. Try to do something that makes you feel good every day to help relieve stress. It doesn't have to take long; even 15 to 20 minutes will suffice. Examples of relaxing hobbies include:

- Reading a novel
- Knitting a cloth
- Working on an art project
- Playing golf in the golf course
- Watching a movie
- Enjoy doing puzzles
- Playing Card and board games

H. Discuss Your Issues

If something is upsetting you, talking about it can help you relax. You can discuss your feelings with family members, friends, a trusted clergyman, your doctor, or a therapist.

You can also converse with yourself. Self-talk is something we all do. However, in order for self-talk to help lower stress, it must be positive rather than negative.

So, when you're stressed, pay close attention to what you're thinking or saying. Change the negative message you're sending yourself to a positive one. Don't tell yourself, for example, "I can't do this." Instead, tell yourself, "I can do this" or "I'm doing my best."

I. Be Gentle With Yourself.

Accept that no matter how hard you try, you will never be able to do everything flawlessly. You also don't have complete control over your life. So, do yourself a favor and stop believing you can accomplish so much. And remember to preserve your sense of humor. Laughter might help you feel more at ease.

J. Get Rid of Your Triggers.

Determine the major sources of stress in your life. Is it your job, your commute, or your studies? If you can determine what they are, see if you can eradicate or at least lessen them from your life.

If you can't pinpoint the root causes of your stress, create a stress journal. Make a note of when you feel the most anxious and see if you can spot a trend; then, discover solutions to eliminate or reduce those triggers.

Building Self-Esteem And Self-Worth

Depression and poor self-esteem are the same thing. While poor self-esteem predisposes people to depression, depression can completely destroy self-esteem.

Even if your poor self-esteem is deeply ingrained, there are things you can do to improve it, even if you are depressed.

A. Establish the tone: Make the most of every morning.

It is critical that you begin each day on a positive note. This will train your mind to notice good qualities—excellent ones—in yourself. So, surround oneself with positive things like music, literature, calendars, computer wallpaper, and so forth. You can even subscribe to a service that will bring you hilarious memes or videos of cute animals every day. Feeling good at the start of the day will set the tone for the rest of the day.

B. Recognize and Correct Negative Self-Talk.

Negative thinking causes both low self-esteem and depression. The more one thinks negatively, the less one is able to understand themselves and the world around them objectively. Soon, the negative ideas become stuck in a loop, like an old record that keeps skipping, causing the same lyric to repeat itself.

C. Start questioning your negative self-talk.

The ability to detect and examine one's own ideas is required first. When you have a self-critical idea, you do not have to believe it. While many thoughts are automatic, learning to manage your own negative thoughts is an essential part of overcoming depression! Here are some questions to consider the next time you have critical thoughts:

- Is there any proof to back this up?

- Where did this idea come from? Is this anything I've heard said before? If so, are they reliable source of knowledge about me?
- Would I ever tell myself that if I were a friend?
- Is this notion making me feel good or horrible about myself?
- Even if this concept is correct, is it beneficial to dwell on it?

When you understand there is no proof to back up your thinking, that your friends and family would disagree with you, and that your thought makes you feel horrible about yourself, it's time to replace it, not with a broad affirmation but with specific, meaningful self-statements.

D. Reframing Negative Thoughts to Combat Depression.

Let's say you have a big project at work or school and are feeling stressed out. "Why did I say I could manage this?" "I was naive to think I could do a good job on this," or "Can things ever get any worse than this?" You might opt to replace such negative thoughts with positive factual ones, such as "I'm getting better at this work every day and am making progress." "I'm a hard worker," you might say. Even when it's challenging, I keep going and try to see things from multiple perspectives.

Being perfect or believing you are flawless when you are not is not a sign of healthy self-esteem. Nobody is. A good sense of self-worth is about recognizing your talents, understanding your weaknesses, and knowing that you are human and delightfully flawed like everyone else. Positive self-talk can assist you in feeling more empowered and confident.

E. Be Kind to Yourself and Take Care of Yourself.

Even if you believe you don't deserve it, treating yourself will send positive messages to your subconscious mind that you are worth it. You could treat yourself to a nice meal, buy that sweater you've been eyeing, or make an appointment for a relaxing massage. You don't even have to spend money; simply spend time reading a book, taking a walk in nature, or doing something that inspires you.

F. Surround yourself with positive people.

You want to be surrounded by people who praise your strengths, not your flaws. Seeking the help of a therapist who can help you look at and change your negative thought patterns is one way to get help. When we don't have an accurate self-perception, getting a fresh view from an objective third party can be beneficial.

It's not easy to boost your self-esteem, but if you follow these techniques, you'll be able to chip away at the negative self-talk every day.

Building A Support Network: How To Find And Connect With People Who Can Help

Getting support is a key part of dealing with anxiety disorders and other mental health problems. Support networks can help you when you need it most by giving you hope, comfort, and practical help. Here are some tips for building a support network:

A. **Connect with people who understand**: Surround yourself with people who understand what you're going through, whether it's through therapy, support groups, or online communities.
B. **Build a trusted circle**: Seek out friends, family members, or professionals who are willing to listen, offer advice, and be there for you in tough times.
C. **Join a support group**: Many communities have local support groups for people with anxiety disorders, or you can find online groups. This can be a great way to connect with others and share experiences.
D. **Turn to friends and family**: Reach out to trusted friends and family members for support and advice. If you don't feel comfortable discussing your anxiety with them, consider seeking the help of a mental health professional.

E. **Volunteer:** Volunteering can be a great way to connect with others and feel a sense of purpose.

F. **Practice self-care**: Taking care of yourself physically, emotionally, and mentally will help you build resilience and cope with stress and anxiety.

G. **Seek professional help**: Mental health professionals can provide individualized support, guidance, and treatment for anxiety disorders. They can help you develop coping skills and offer strategies for managing stress and worry.

Building a support network is an important step in managing anxiety disorders. Surrounding yourself with people who care and who understand what you're going through can help you feel more supported and less isolated.

Seven Anxiety Support Groups

What precisely are anxiety support groups?

Anxiety support groups give people the chance to get together regularly with others who are going through similar feelings and situations and can help each other.

To alleviate feelings of loneliness, members can share their experiences and coping skills.

The medium of support differs depending on the platform. Many feature free and anonymous internet discussion forums. Some companies provide virtual meetings or one-on-one chat rooms for real-time help from home.

Online anxiety support groups and online group therapy sessions are ideal for people who do not have access to other mental health services or who want to supplement their current treatment.

These groups can also benefit those who have successfully managed their anxiety symptoms and want to help others.

A. **Support Groups Central:** Overall best

How to join: Joining is free, although certain meetings have a nominal fee.

Advantages: Meetings are led by trained teachers (using the microphone and camera is optional)

Disadvantages: Some meetings have a small fee, and you can't chat with text.

Means of Support: Support comes in the form of video and audio calls.

Target Audience: For individuals looking for meetings that are easily accessible, confidential, and instructor-led.

This is described as "a place where people can gather to help and encourage one another with a range of life challenges."

Support Groups Central, which is available globally, assists people from over 120 nations. Members can join via video and audio, and they can remain anonymous by turning off the camera and entering a username.

The meetings are led by training instructors. Many of them are certified, licensed, or hold advanced degrees in their fields. Each instructor must complete and pass the Support Groups Central video-based meeting training program.

According to the website, 95% of users would recommend Support Groups Central to others. Users report fewer symptoms, less use of emergency symptoms, and fewer hospital stays.

B. **Anxiety and Depression Association of America:** Best forum for online discussion

Price: Free.

Advantages: It is owned by a highly renowned organization and is controlled by administrators.

Disadvantages: The absence of trained specialists.

Types Of Support: Discussion forums

Target Audience: For people looking for peer-to-peer support through online chat-based discussion forums

The Anxiety and Depression Association of America (ADAA) focuses on the treatment of anxiety and depression. ADAA uses evidence-based programs, such as online anxiety support groups, to improve the quality of life for people who are getting help for their mental health.

The website provides free peer-to-peer support groups where people can share knowledge and experiences in online chat rooms. There is also a section in Spanish.

Support is not coordinated by skilled specialists. The community is overseen by administrators, and members must follow the rules.

Users say that the online group is an easy and safe way to connect with other people who are feeling the same way. Users are at different points in their mental health journeys, so helping those who need it the most gives some of them a sense of satisfaction.

While the online community is not intended to replace emergency medical services or professional mental health services, it does provide a safe environment for people suffering from anxiety and depression to talk with others who understand.

C. Mental Health America: Best for unlimited access

Cost: Free

Advantages: There are free mental health screening tests, which are like a social network for mental health.

Disadvantages: Non-members can view posts and other activity.

Means of Support: Support comes in the form of a discussion forum.

Target Audience: For those who want constant access to a community of people who share their thoughts and feelings.

Mental Health America is a community-based, non-profit organization dedicated to providing mental health services for prevention, intervention, and treatment.

The Inspire-hosted Mental Health America online support group is a free place for people with anxiety, depression, and other mental health problems to ask questions, share their experiences, and get help from a community that understands.

This group operates on a peer-to-peer basis and is moderated by group leaders. To see if you have symptoms of a mental health condition, the organization provides free mental health screening tests, including one for anxiety.

D. **SMART Recovery:** This is ideal for people who are also dealing with addiction.

Cost: Free

Advantages: Access to scientific resources for tackling harmful behaviors and promoting long-term change

Disadvantages: The emphasis is on addiction rather than anxiety.

Means of support: Support is available in the form of in-person and online meetings, as well as online discussion boards.

Target Audience: For people who suffer from anxiety as well as addiction

SMART Recovery provides assistance to people suffering from addiction and other detrimental habits.

While the techniques and resources are not specifically aimed at anxiety, they are useful for people who want to maintain effective long-term change or those who suffer from anxiety and addiction.

If you use mental health resources to deal with your anxiety, SMART Recovery may be able to help. You set your own pace, whether you follow the programs or attend the meetings.

"SMART is not just any mutual-help program," according to the website. "Our science-based approach stresses self-reliance and empowerment."

Meetings are held both in-person and online, giving members the option to choose based on their preferences and availability.

View the calendar for online meetings and events to attend a SMART Recovery meeting. Registration is free, and you will have access to over 40 online meetings per week.

Members also have access to free online discussion boards 24 hours a day, seven days a week.

E. 7 Cups: The Best Anxiety Support App

Price: While the 24/7 chat rooms, discussion forums, and app are free, professional counseling is not.

Advantages: The listeners have been trained.

Disadvantages: New users do not have immediate access to all functions.

Means of Support: Support options include private one-on-one chat rooms, discussion forums, and group gatherings.

Target Audience: For people seeking assistance from their devices.

7 Cups regard themselves as "the world's largest emotional support system." You may get help from your smartphone by downloading

the free app. It is available for download from the Apple App Store and the Google Play Store.

7 Cups connects people with professional listeners to provide free emotional assistance. You can talk one-on-one with a listener in a private chat room or join one of the 7 Cups online communities, which include an anxiety support community.

Every week, 7 Cups hosts dozens of free online events, such as support groups and sharing circles.

According to 7 Cups research, 90% of people feel better after speaking with listeners, and 80% believe listeners can help people with mental health difficulties.

F. **SupportGroups.com**: Good for those interested in joining multiple groups

Cost: Free

Advantages: Groups are extremely specialized.

Disadvantages: The group is not as highly moderated as others.

Means of Support: Discussion forums are one type of help.

Target Audience: For people looking for anxiety and other topic support groups.

SupportGroups.com is a free online support group hub with an anxiety group with over 100,000 members.

The website has a list of resources to help people find the specialized care they need, as well as a regularly updated blog with suggestions about mental health.

Members can post anonymously in the discussion areas regarding anxiety, self-esteem, loneliness, and other topics. Other members can interact with and comment on postings to uplift and connect with those who are going through similar emotions and experiences.

This is a great alternative if you want to join a number of online support groups. However, it does not appear that the site is as well monitored as others.

G. **TheTribe:** Ideal for anxiety-relieving activities.

Cost: Free

Advantages: It has a wide community and a toolbox of anxiety-relieving resources.

Disadvantages: Not designed expressly for anxiety.

Means of Support: Chat rooms and discussion forums

Target Audience: People who are looking for resources like mood charts, uplifting activities, and other tools, as well as support groups for anxiety.

TheTribe provides peer support groups for people suffering from addiction, anxiety, depression, HIV, and obsessive-compulsive disorder. Other organizations exist for members of the LGBTQIA+ community, people who are married and raising families, and teenagers.

The website also provides information for anyone in need of internet treatment.

According to TheTribe, "Members of our support groups have discovered that, in addition to professional therapy, sharing stories and meeting others with anxiety can be therapeutic."

TheTribe professes to be more than just a support group. In addition to online communities, TheTribe provides a supportive and encouraging environment. Members are encouraged to do things that are fun and inspiring, connect with other people, keep track of their mood, and more.

TheTribe is a big community of people who understand, with over 130,000 tribe members.

Tabular Description

Support Groups	Price	Means of Support	Target Audience
Support Groups Central	Free, though some meetings comes with nominal fee	Video and audio calls	For individuals looking for meetings that are easily accessible, confidential, and instructor-led
Anxiety and Depression Association Of America	Free	Discussion forums	For people looking for peer-to-peer support through online chat-based discussion forums
Mental Health America	Free	Discussion community	For those who want constant access to a community of people who share their thoughts and feelings
SMART Recovery	Free	In-person meetings; Online meetings; Online discussions.	For people who suffer from anxiety as well as addiction
7 Cups	Free for App, Chat rooms and discussion groups; Professional therapy is an additional cost.	Discussion forums; Group meetings; One-on-one chat rooms	For people seeking assistance from their devices.
SupportGroups.com	Free	Discussion forums	for people looking for anxiety and other topic support groups.
TheTribe	Free	Discussion forums Chat rooms	for individuals seeking resources such as mood charts, uplifting activities, and other tools, as well as anxiety support groups.

How To Communicate Effectively With Loved Ones And Friends

Effective communication with loved ones and friends is crucial in building a strong support network and managing anxiety. Theto following are some tips for effective communication:

A. **Be Clear and Direct**: Be clear and direct in your communication. Explain what you need and what you are feeling.
B. **Listen actively**: Listen to the other person's perspective and try to understand their point of view.
C. **Avoid Blaming**: Avoid blaming others for your problems and instead focus on finding solutions together.
D. **Use "I" Statements**: Use "I" statements to express your feelings, rather than making accusations. For example, instead of saying "you always make me feel bad," say "I feel bad when I feel ignored."
E. **Be Open and Honest**: Be open and honest about your feelings and what you need from the relationship.
F. **Practice Empathy**: Try to put yourself in the other person's shoes and understand their perspective.
G. **Avoid Arguing**: If a disagreement arises, try to avoid arguing and instead focus on finding a solution that works for both parties.
H. **Take Responsibility**: Take responsibility for your own feelings and actions and avoid blaming others.

By following these tips, you can communicate effectively with your loved ones and friends, build a strong support network, and better manage anxiety.

How to Communicate Effectively with a Therapist or Counselor

Effective communication with a therapist or counselor is important in order to get the most benefit from therapy. When you can clearly and openly express your thoughts and feelings, your therapist can better understand your needs and tailor their approach to help you. Here are some tips on how to communicate effectively with a therapist:

A. **Be honest and open**: Be honest and open with your therapist about what you are feeling and what you need help with. If you are feeling nervous, overwhelmed or anything else, let them know.

B. **Ask questions**: If you don't understand something your therapist is saying, don't hesitate to ask for clarification. The goal is for you to understand and be comfortable with the therapy process.

C. **Share your thoughts and feelings**: Your therapist is there to help you work through your feelings and thoughts, so it is important to share them openly and honestly. This can be difficult, but it is a crucial part of the therapy process.

D. **Set goals**: Together with your therapist, set goals for what you want to achieve from therapy. This can help you stay focused and motivated during the process.

E. **Provide feedback**: Let your therapist know if their approach is helpful or not. This can help them tailor their approach to better meet your needs.

F. **Be open to change**: The therapy process can be challenging and may involve change, but it is important to be open to the process and embrace the changes that may come.

By following these tips, you can communicate effectively with your therapist and get the most out of your therapy sessions.

How To Communicate Effectively With A Doctor Or Other Medical Professional

Effective communication with a doctor or other medical professional is critical to managing anxiety disorders and getting the best care. Here are some tips for improving communication with medical professionals:

A. **Be clear about your symptoms and concerns**: Make a list of all the symptoms you are experiencing and share them with your doctor. If you are unsure about what's causing your anxiety, be open about that as well.

B. **Ask questions**: Don't be afraid to ask questions and seek clarification. If you don't understand something, it's better to ask for an explanation than to leave with misconceptions.

C. **Be honest**: Tell your doctor about any previous treatments you've tried and their effectiveness. Also, let them know if there are any lifestyle changes you've made to manage your anxiety, such as exercise or mindfulness practices.

D. **Be specific**: Give specific examples of your symptoms and how they affect your daily life. This helps the doctor get a better understanding of what you're going through.

E. **Bring a trusted friend or family member**: Having someone you trust with you during the appointment can help you feel more confident and less anxious. They can also help you remember important details from the appointment.

F. **Take notes**: It's a good idea to bring a notebook and pen with you to take notes during the appointment. This helps you remember the doctor's recommendations and any new information you learn.

By following these tips, you can improve your communication with your doctor and get the most out of your appointments. Effective communication can help you get a better diagnosis and treatment, which will help you deal with your anxiety disorder in the long run.

SETTING GOALS AND CREATING A PLAN TO MANAGE ANXIETY

Setting goals and creating a plan is an important step in managing an anxiety disorder. This involves identifying the specific symptoms or behaviors that are causing the most distress and determining what steps can be taken to reduce or eliminate these symptoms. The steps below can help you come up with a good plan for dealing with anxiety:

A. **Identify the specific symptoms**: Write down the specific symptoms or behaviors that are causing the most distress, such as panic attacks, excessive worry, physical symptoms, etc.

B. **Assess the impact of the symptoms**: Consider how the symptoms are affecting your daily life, such as work, relationships, and activities.

C. **Set achievable goals**: Determine what you want to achieve, and set achievable and realistic goals. For example, if you suffer from panic attacks, your goal may be to reduce the frequency and severity of the attacks.

D. **Choose strategies and techniques.** Based on the specific symptoms and goals, choose strategies and techniques that have been shown to help manage anxiety, such as cognitive-behavioral therapy (CBT), exposure therapy, mindfulness, relaxation techniques, medication, and self-help resources.

E. **Create a plan**: Write down the specific steps you will take to achieve your goals, and set a timeline for each step. This could include attending therapy sessions, practicing relaxation techniques, adjusting your diet and exercise routine, and reaching out to support networks.

F. **Monitor progress**: Keep track of your progress, and adjust your plan as needed. If you are not making progress, consider seeking the help of a professional.

G. **Build resilience**: Build resilience by engaging in self-care activities, such as exercise, sleep, and healthy eating. Find ways to cultivate positive thinking, such as practicing gratitude and mindfulness.

H. **Reach out for support**: Connect with loved ones, friends, and support groups to build a support network. Reach out to your therapist or doctor for guidance and support when needed.

By setting goals and creating a plan, you can take control of your anxiety disorder, reduce the impact of symptoms, and improve your overall quality of life.

Understanding The Importance Of Goal-Setting For Managing Anxiety

Setting goals is an important part of dealing with anxiety because it gives you a sense of direction, motivation, and control. It enables people to focus on what they want to accomplish rather than being controlled by their anxiety. Setting specific, achievable, and realistic goals can help individuals break down the process of managing their anxiety into smaller, more manageable steps. This makes it easier to track progress and see the results of their efforts. Additionally, setting goals provides a sense of accomplishment and boosts self-confidence, which can help reduce anxiety levels.

A well-crafted goal should be clear, measurable, and time-bound. It should also be aligned with an individual's values and priorities. For example, a goal for managing anxiety might be "To reduce my panic attacks from once a week to once a month by the end of the year." This goal is clear, measurable, and has a deadline because it sets a goal for reducing panic attacks in a certain amount of time.

Having a goal in place can also provide a sense of purpose and focus, which can help individuals stay motivated even when they face challenges. Setting goals can also help people figure out how to deal with their anxiety and give them a clear picture of what they want to achieve. In turn, this can help reduce stress and worry and increase a sense of control and self-efficacy.

How To Set Realistic And Achievable Goals For Managing Anxiety

Setting goals might help you overcome some aspects of anxiety disorders. Here are some tips to help you set goals for your anxiety problem and reach them.

The Most Effective Goals

The term "S.M.A.R.T." is frequently used in relation to goal setting.

S.M.A.R.T. is an acronym that stands for:

- Specific
- Measurable
- Achievable
- Realistic
- Time-Bound

For example, you may set a goal of making five new acquaintances this year.

Your objective is **specific** (5 friends), **measurable** (whether it is possible for you to hit this aim), **achievable** (if you work hard at meeting new people), **realistic** (many people have at least 5 friends), and **time-bound** (to be achieved in the next 12 months).

An unreasonable objective would be to never experience anxiety in social or performance situations. Such black-and-white thinking sets you up for failure because you will almost always feel anxious in those situations.

Here are some excellent steps for setting objectives:

A. Determine your objectives.

What would you like to change about your anxiety problems? Select short-, medium-, and long-term objectives in areas such as:

- Making new acquaintances
- Finding work

- Getting physically fit

Don't let your nervousness get in the way of setting goals. Identify goals, regardless of how anxious they may make you feel.

Make a list of your goals to ensure that you stick to them.

B. Divide your goals into manageable bits.

For example, if your goal is to make one phone call per day, begin by deciding who you will call and double-checking that you have the correct phone number.

C. Identify potential roadblocks.

What might stand in your way of establishing five new friends? Identify the difficulties and devise solutions to overcome them. If you don't see others very often, join a club or take some form of class to meet new people.

D. Establish goals.

Make regular time to work toward your objective. In the case of making five new acquaintances, plan regular activities that will bring you into contact with potential pals. For example, you could go to the gym at the same time every week in the hopes of seeing the same people.

E. Complete your objective.

It is possible that you may need to write down the exact measures you will take to reach your goal. For the new friends, this could involve jotting down things like conversation starters, how to keep the conversation going, and so on.

Goal-Achieving Motivation

Having goals to work on your anxiety problem will not help if you are still unmotivated.

Identify and tackle the blockages that keep you from feeling motivated, such as believing things will never change.

Reward or Revise Your Goals

If you have achieved your objectives, reward yourself. If not, modify to improve your chances of succeeding the next time.

Identifying Triggers And Warning Signs Of Anxiety

Identifying triggers and warning signs of anxiety is an important step in managing the condition. Triggers are events, situations, or thoughts that can set off anxiety symptoms. They are unique to each individual and can vary from person to person. Some common triggers include stress at work, financial worries, relationship issues, health problems, or a traumatic event.

Warning signs of anxiety can include physical symptoms such as sweating, increased heart rate, muscle tension, fatigue, and trouble sleeping. There can also be emotional symptoms such as feelings of worry, fear, and nervousness, as well as behavioral symptoms such as avoidance of certain situations, excessive worry, and repetitive behaviors.

By recognizing your triggers and warning signs, you can be better prepared to manage your anxiety. This can involve developing coping strategies to help you deal with triggers, seeking support from friends or a therapist, practicing relaxation techniques, or making lifestyle changes such as exercise or a change in diet.

Identifying triggers and warning signs is also important in creating a plan to manage anxiety. This plan can include setting goals, seeking support, developing coping strategies, and making positive lifestyle changes. With the right support and resources, it is possible to manage anxiety and lead a fulfilling life.

How To Develop A Plan For Managing Anxiety

Developing a plan for managing anxiety involves several steps:

A. **Understanding your anxiety**: Start by identifying your specific anxiety disorder, the symptoms, and triggers. Keep a journal of your symptoms and when they occur.

B. **Setting goals**: Set specific, measurable, attainable, relevant, and time-bound (SMART) goals to work towards managing your anxiety.

C. **Developing coping strategies**: Identify healthy coping mechanisms that work for you, such as exercise, mindfulness, or deep breathing.

D. **Creating a support network**: Surround yourself with people who can provide support and encouragement. This can include friends, family, or a support group.

E. **Taking action**: Take small, gradual steps towards achieving your goals and practicing your coping strategies. Be patient and persistent, as change can take time.

F. **Reviewing progress**: Regularly evaluate your progress and adjust your plan as needed. Celebrate your accomplishments and acknowledge any setbacks as opportunities to learn and grow.

G. **Seeking professional help**: If you're struggling to manage your anxiety on your own, consider reaching out to a mental health professional for support. A therapist can help you develop an effective treatment plan and provide additional tools for managing anxiety.

Remember, everyone's journey to managing anxiety is different. It's important to find what works for you and be consistent in your approach. With time and effort, you can learn to manage your anxiety and lead a more fulfilling life.

How To Prioritize And Balance Competing Demands

Balancing competing demands is a common challenge in today's fast-paced world. It can be especially hard for people with anxiety, because stress and pressure from many different places can make them feel and think anxious. Prioritizing tasks and responsibilities based on how important they are and how quickly they need to be done can help you deal with competing demands and reduce stress. Here are a few tips for prioritizing and balancing competing demands:

A. **Make a list**: Write down all of your tasks and responsibilities, and prioritize them based on importance and urgency.
B. **Set realistic goals**: Be realistic about what you can achieve in a given day or week, and set achievable goals for yourself.
C. **Prioritize self-care**: Make sure to include self-care activities such as exercise, meditation, and relaxation in your daily routine.
D. **Delegate tasks**: When possible, delegate tasks to others, especially those that are not critical or that can be done by someone else.
E. **Use time-management strategies**: Utilize tools such as calendars, timers, and to-do lists to stay organized and on track.
F. **Learn to say NO**: It's okay to decline requests or responsibilities that will overburden you or cause undue stress.
G. **Create boundaries**: Set clear boundaries between work and personal life, and make time for activities that bring joy and relaxation.

By prioritizing tasks, setting realistic goals, and taking care of yourself, you can balance competing demands and reduce stress and anxiety.

How To Monitor Progress And Adjust The Plan As Needed

Monitoring progress and making changes to the plan as needed are important parts of dealing with anxiety in a healthy way. This means figuring out how well the strategies and techniques you've been using to deal with your anxiety are working and making changes as needed. To do this, it is helpful to keep track of your symptoms, stress levels, and overall wellbeing in a journal or other record-keeping system. Then, you can use this information to find patterns and possible triggers and make changes to your strategy. This could mean changing how often or how hard you exercise or practice mindfulness, or getting more help or advice from a therapist or support group. By checking in on your progress often and making changes as needed, you can help make sure that your plan is still working and helping you deal with your anxiety.

How To Create A Self-Care Plan

The stress and uncertainty of everyday life can make it hard to stick to a self-care routine. According to a new Birchbox poll, one in every three people feels bad for taking time for themselves, although the majority wishes they did.

Some people regard self-care as a selfish act. In actuality, the inverse is true. When you take care of your physical, emotional, and mental health, you and the people in your life would gain significantly.

Learn why self-care is important for your health and how to design your own individual self-care plan.

What Exactly Is A Self-Care Plan

A self-care plan is a collection of everyday activities that we intentionally engage in to promote our inner and outer well-being. Self-care is more than just pampering and grooming yourself, although that is a component of it.

We take care of our holistic wellbeing—our mental, emotional, and physical health—by following a self-care regimen. We can live healthier, happier, and more fulfilled lives if we take time every day to care for all parts of ourselves.

Self-care plans are a lifelong journey that differs from individual to individual. This is because everyone has a unique set of physical and emotional requirements that must be met. You might feel refreshed after a hard workout, but someone else might like to meditate instead. Strategies for self-care that work for you may not work for someone else.

Self-care programs also keep you from picking up bad habits and teach you how to deal with stressful situations and events in your life.

5 Reasons Why You Need A Self-Care Strategy

A well-planned self-care regimen improves your general well-being. Here are five good reasons why everyone should have one:

A. Promotes better mental health and well-being.

Making time for self-care activities that offer you joy and help you relax is good for your mental health and well-being.

Connecting with others and engaging in daily exercise are simple yet powerful strategies to maintain a positive state of mind. Regular exercise releases compounds that increase your mood, such as endorphins and serotonin. It also boosts your memory and helps you think more clearly.

Mindfulness and learning a new language are two examples of self-care activities that can train your mind. They can assist you in developing your mental fitness, which can improve your mental health and prevent mental fatigue.

B. Deals With Stress And Anxiety

Many of us are subjected to stress on a daily basis. Stress increases the likelihood of developing:

- Anxiety
- Depression
- Workplace exhaustion

When it comes to dealing with stress and anxiety, developing a self-care plan is crucial. It also makes it easier to deal with the symptoms of depression.

The parasympathetic nervous system is stimulated when we exercise self-care. This allows us to unwind both our brains and bodies. Some of the best stress-reduction self-care techniques, according to Dr. Herbert Benson, head of the Benson-Henry Institute for Mind and Body Medicine, are:

- Deep Abdominal breathing

- Yoga
- Visualization
- Tai chi

C. It Keeps You Healthy

Taking care of your mind and body might help you avoid health problems including heart disease, stroke, and cancer. Getting heart disease can be avoided by not smoking and drinking less alcohol.

A constant self-care routine also helps to maintain your general physical wellness. The World Health Organization (WHO) says that self-care is "the ability of individuals, families, and communities to promote health, prevent disease, and keep health."

The more you participate in activities that encourage excellent hygiene, a healthy diet, and an active lifestyle, the more likely you are to avoid disease and boost your immune system.

D. Increases Productivity

Productivity is frequently confused with getting as much done as possible. As a result, self-care is put to the side to make room for working more and doing more until you burn out.

Prioritizing self-care, on the other hand, is the key to becoming more productive at home and at work. According to Dr. Russell Thackeray, a registered clinical psychologist, people who practice self-care have improved cognitive capacities, including improved focus and concentration. As a result, they have a tendency to generate more.

When you give yourself exactly what you need to function at your peak, your work performance will improve automatically.

E. It Improves Personal Ties.

One of the most popular misconceptions about self-care is that it is an act of selfishness. It's no surprise that Americans avoid me-time since it makes them feel guilty. According to Birchbox, two-thirds of Americans prioritize their well-being over caring for others and social responsibility.

But how can you fill other people's cups if your own is empty? Making time to be kind to yourself is not at all selfish. It improves your abilities as a friend, caregiver, coworker, or love partner. Bringing your best self to a relationship deepens your bond with the people around you.

You can also incorporate your loved ones into your self-care strategy. Going for a daily walk with a friend, for example, is a terrific way to bond while also practicing self-care.

The Most Important Factors Of Self-Care

Self-care feeds the mind, body, and spirit. Let's look at some of the most significant aspects of wellbeing and how we might incorporate them into our self-care strategy.

A. Physical.

Physical self-care entails making lifestyle choices that keep you fit, healthy, and energized. Here's how to take care of your physical health:

- Exercise on a daily basis.
- Take walks in nature.
- Maintain regular visits with your medical providers.
- Consume a nutrient-dense, well-balanced diet.
- Maintain a healthy circadian rhythm by practicing appropriate sleeping habits.
- Stop smoking.
- Consume in moderation.
- Get enough rest.

Physical self-care entails developing healthy behaviors that improve your well-being and eliminating unhealthy ones.

B. Mental

This aspect of self-care is all about taking care of your mental health. In other words, it is important to take care of your thoughts and feelings. How you talk to yourself and what you tell yourself has a big effect on how you see yourself and the rest of the world.

Mental self-care also entails mental training. You must exercise your mind in the same way that you train your body. A sharp intellect allows you to better deal with stress and navigate major life changes.

These mental self-care practices can assist you in keeping your mind healthy and sharp:

- Spend meaningful time with family and friends.
- Set professional objectives.
- Discover something new.
- Take up an activity that you enjoy.
- Give your phone a break.
- Use positive self-talk.

C. Emotional

Emotional well-being is about becoming more aware of our emotional needs by paying attention to how we feel. This helps us deal with our feelings in a healthy way, by focusing on the good and dealing with the bad.

Let's look at some effective techniques to boost your mental health:

- Meditate.
- Begin keeping a journal.
- Exercise self-compassion.
- Observe your ideas without passing judgment.
- Exercise thankfulness.
- Breathing exercises might help you regulate your emotions.
- Perform acts of compassion.

Emotional self-care allows you to respond to life's problems rather than react to them. Responding implies that you address an issue with caution and consideration. On the other hand, reacting is an emotional response that often has a bad effect.

D. Professional

Professional self-care is any action that helps you do well at work while keeping a healthy balance between work and life.

Self-care in the workplace might include activities that help you improve professionally and give you a sense of fulfillment, such as practicing inner work or applying for a promotion.

Here are some further occupational self-care practices:

- Make the most of your vacation time.
- Prior to meetings, make time for yourself.
- Develop a new soft skill.
- Work for a company that values employee well-being.
- Turn into a mentor.

There are five phases to creating a self-care strategy.

The best self-care plan for you is one that is tailored to your specific requirements. Begin your unique self-care regimen right away by doing the following:

a. Examine Your Current Habits.

Examine your current situation before developing a strategy for self-care. What tactics do you employ to deal with life's challenges?

Do you go for a stroll to reduce stress, or do you isolate yourself from friends and family? Do you drink a few too many glasses of wine after a long day at work, or do you take a lengthy bath to unwind?

Make an honest inventory of the positive and negative coping methods you've built over time. This step helps you figure out your bad habits and how you currently take care of yourself.

b. Determine Your Self-Care Requirements.

Consider what you value most in your daily life. Create a list of your physical, mental, emotional, and professional requirements. A self-care plan that covers all aspects of well-being is an excellent example.

Writing down your wants and requirements can be eye-opening. You might find that you are taking care of your physical needs but not your emotional ones.

c. Make A List Of Practices That Will Help You Meet Your Needs.

Now you must pick which self-care activities will best help you meet your needs. Consider asking yourself the following questions:

- What hobbies make me happy?
- What gives me a boost of energy?
- When do I feel most at ease?
- What gives me a sense of accomplishment?
- What has helped me get through difficult times in my life?

Write down the self-care routines you intend to conduct on a regular basis as well as those you intend to do just sometimes. For example, you may wish to eat healthy every day but only have supper with a friend once a week.

d. Make Room For Them In Your Calendar.

Now comes the difficult part. You must schedule time for these practices throughout your busy day. Remember that self-care is not a selfish act. It's an act of self-compassion.

Instead of cramming everything into your day, start small. Making a significant change may feel daunting, forcing you to abandon your goal. Instead, incorporate one to two new things into your weekly schedule.

Begin with the ones you require and value the most and work your way down. Your priorities will shift from time to time as well. When you have a cold, for example, your bodily requirements take priority over professional self-care.

Evaluate how these self-care routines are benefiting you and add more to your plan as you go.

e. Remove Any Impediments

Remember those bad habits you mentioned earlier? It's time to say goodbye. These self-destructive coping mechanisms are impeding your self-care plan.

Begin by lowering and then eliminating unhealthy coping behaviors. Choose the most harmful one and replace it with a self-care habit.

Don't be afraid to ask your friends or family for assistance. Sharing your plan for self-care with people who care about you will make it easier to get past problems.

How To Keep To Your Self-Care Routine

It takes time and consistency for a self-care plan to work.

Keep your strategy simple and select self-care activities that you enjoy. The secret to adhering to your routine is to do activities that make you happy.

Your self-care strategy can also be as adaptable as you require. You will have good days and bad days. When things don't go as planned, don't be too hard on yourself. A new start is always possible.

How To Create A Crisis Plan

A crisis plan is a set of strategies and actions that can be taken in the event of an emergency or crisis situation to help manage symptoms of anxiety. The goal of a crisis plan is to give the person a plan for how to deal with anxiety symptoms and make sure they have the tools and support they need to deal with their anxiety well. A crisis plan should include the following:

A. **Triggers and warning signs of anxiety**: Identifying the specific situations, thoughts, or events that trigger anxiety symptoms.
B. **Coping strategies**: Listing the specific coping strategies that have worked in the past, such as deep breathing, mindfulness, or physical exercise.

C. **Support network**: Identifying the people who can provide support and assistance during a crisis, such as friends, family, or a therapist.
D. **Emergency contact information**: Keeping a list of emergency contacts, including a doctor, therapist, or crisis helpline.
E. **Self-care**: Making a list of activities that can help to manage anxiety symptoms, such as meditation, reading, or listening to music.
F. **Medications**: Keeping a list of medications that are taken for anxiety, including dosage and frequency.
G. **Crisis plan review**: Regularly reviewing and updating the crisis plan to ensure that it remains relevant and effective.

It is important to share the crisis plan with trusted family members, friends, or a therapist so that they can provide support and assistance if needed.

How To Create A Plan For Maintaining Long-Term Recovery

Maintaining long-term recovery from anxiety disorder requires ongoing effort and commitment. It's important to make a plan for dealing with anxiety that covers the physical, emotional, and mental parts. Some strategies for maintaining long-term recovery include:

A. **Continuing therapy or counseling**: Regular sessions with a mental health professional can help individuals identify and address any challenges that arise.
B. **Practicing stress-management techniques**: Techniques such as mindfulness, deep breathing, and progressive muscle relaxation can help individuals manage stress and reduce symptoms of anxiety.
C. **Exercising regularly**: Regular exercise can help improve physical and mental health and reduce symptoms of anxiety.
D. **Eating a healthy diet**: A balanced and nutritious diet can help individuals feel their best and manage symptoms of anxiety.

E. **Staying connected**: Building and maintaining strong relationships with friends, family, and support groups can provide a sense of belonging and support.

F. **Monitoring triggers**: Keeping track of what triggers symptoms of anxiety and avoiding or modifying these triggers can help maintain long-term recovery.

G. **Seeking professional help when needed**: If symptoms of anxiety become severe or persistent, it may be necessary to seek professional help.

By putting these strategies into a comprehensive plan, people with anxiety disorder can build resilience and keep getting better over time. It's important to remember that recovery is a journey and that it's okay to ask for help and support along the way.

How To Create A Plan For Relapse Prevention

Relapse prevention is an important part of treating anxiety disorders because it keeps people who have made a lot of progress in their recovery from going backwards. To create a plan for relapse prevention, the following steps can be taken:

A. **Identify triggers and warning signs:** This means learning what things and situations, like stress, fatigue, or trauma, can cause an episode of anxiety. This can help you prepare for these situations and reduce the likelihood of a relapse.

B. **Create a coping plan**: Once you have identified your triggers, it is important to have a plan for coping with them when they arise. This can involve engaging in stress-management techniques, seeking support from others, or using relaxation exercises.

C. **Develop a support network**: Building a support network of friends, family, and professionals can be essential in preventing relapse. Having people to turn to when you need support can be instrumental in helping you manage anxiety.

D. **Stay engaged in treatment**: Regular therapy sessions, medication management, and other forms of treatment can help keep anxiety under control and prevent relapse.

E. **Practice self-care**: Engaging in self-care activities such as exercise, mindfulness, and healthy eating can help manage symptoms of anxiety and prevent relapse.

F. **Set realistic goals**: Setting realistic, achievable goals can help keep you motivated and focused on maintaining your recovery.

G. **Monitor your progress**: Regularly monitoring your progress and assessing how well your plan is working can help you make any necessary adjustments. If you notice that a particular aspect of your plan is not working, make changes to ensure that it is more effective.

By following these steps, people can make a complete plan to prevent relapse, which can help them stay free of anxiety disorders for the long term.

IDENTIFYING AND AVOIDING RELAPSE TRIGGERS

Relapse triggers are events, situations, or thoughts that can cause a person to return to a previous state of anxiety or to start experiencing anxiety again. It's important to identify these triggers as part of a plan for relapse prevention.

Examples of common relapse triggers include:

- **Stressful life events**: Such as a breakup, job loss, financial difficulties, or illness.
- **Substance use**: Substance abuse can trigger anxiety and is also a common trigger for relapse.
- **Unresolved conflicts**: Such as conflicts with a partner, family member, or friend.
- **Negative thoughts**: Such as worry, rumination, and negative self-talk.
- **Lifestyle changes**: Such as changes in sleeping patterns, exercise habits, or eating habits.

Once you know what sets you off, you can make plans to avoid or deal with them. For example, you can use relaxation techniques to manage stress or seek support from a trusted friend or therapist to help you navigate conflicts. You can also practice cognitive-behavioral therapy (CBT) techniques to challenge and change negative thoughts.

It's also important to develop a plan for what to do if you experience a relapse. This can mean going to a therapist or support group, taking better care of yourself, and refocusing on your goals and progress.

Triggers Of Relapse And How To Avoid Them

It is not uncommon for people in recovery from addictions to relapse at least once. Some people even go off the wagon multiple times before finally getting sober for good. In fact, despite FDA-approved treatments for nicotine, alcohol, and opioid addiction, more than two-thirds of those who begin treatment will relapse.

Understanding what can cause you to relapse and having a plan in place to deal with these triggers are the first steps toward prevention. Here are five triggers to think about and discuss with your therapist or counselor.

A. Stress

The leading cause of relapse is stress. Furthermore, many people who struggle with addiction use their substance or activity of choice as a maladaptive coping mechanism. In fact, research shows that under stressful conditions, there is an increased "wanting" for the drug, alcohol, or addictive activity—especially if the substance or activity was the person's major coping technique.

One way to get ready for this trigger is to figure out how stressed you are right now. Although you can't get rid of everyone and everything in your life, you can avoid situations that bring you a lot of stress. As a result, making a list of all the people, places, and things that cause you stress may be beneficial.

For example, are you in a poisonous relationship or dealing with a financial situation that is causing you stress?

You might be able to reduce the amount of stress in your life by changing your habits, relationships, and priorities. And if you do that, stress is less likely to cause you to go back to using.

It is also critical to acquire good stress management techniques.

You may be able to lessen or manage your stress by doing the following:

- Practicing mindfulness and relaxation techniques.
- Improve your time management skills to prevent functioning in panic mode.
- Increasing healthy behaviors through moderate exercise and nutritious nutrition.

Reducing the risk that stress will trigger a relapse requires not just developing healthy methods to deal with stress but also being able to recognize and respond to stressful situations.

A therapist or counselor may help you learn how to listen to your mind and body to figure out when you're stressed and come up with good ways to deal with it.

B. People Or Locations Associated With The Addictive Behavior.

People who were involved in your addictive activity are possible relapse triggers, whether or not they are still drinking, smoking, or taking drugs. Similarly, places that remind you of your addiction can be triggering. Even family members might be a trigger, particularly if they make you feel childish and defenseless.

When you're reminded of your addiction, it's important to have good ways to deal with it. For example, if you're an alcoholic and a group of drinking buddies invite you out or you observe coworkers going to happy hour, having a specific reaction prepared may be beneficial.

It may also be beneficial to have a healthy activity to do instead, such as going for a run, watching a movie, having dinner with a sponsor, or reading a nice book.

You are more likely to relapse if you do not plan ahead of time for these scenarios. Try brainstorming ideas or collaborating with your counselor or therapist to develop a plan.

C. Negative Or Difficult Emotions

Addicts need effective ways to endure, deal with, and make sense of the bad things that happen to them on a regular basis. You can no longer rely on alcohol, drugs, or addictive habits to bring you brief comfort from those feelings.

Learn to be comfortable with unpleasant feelings and emotions.

Recognize that your bad feelings do not have to be an indication of an approaching setback. Everyone experiences negative or difficult feelings. The trick is in how you handle them.

Consider these feelings as a chance for personal development and comprehension. Taking an inventory of your feelings and asking yourself why can teach you a lot about yourself. In fact, understanding how to deal with your emotions without succumbing to addiction is priceless.

When you're feeling down, consider journaling, meditating, or even praying. Find a healthy approach to letting go of negativity and improving your mood. With the help of an addictions specialist or another mental health professional, you can come up with more ways to deal with your problem.

D. Seeing or Sensing the Object of Your Addiction

Reminding yourself of your addiction can lead to relapse throughout recovery. In the early stages of quitting, a whiff of cigarette smoke, seeing people sip cocktails in a bar or restaurant, or seeing a couple locked in a passionate embrace are all reminders.

It is normal to want to return to your addiction. After all, it is a place you are comfortable with. However, recovery involves more than just "quitting" and "abstaining"; it is also about creating a new life in which it is easier—and more desirable—not to use.

Concentrate on the new life you're creating and the improvements you're implementing. Consider the negative consequences of your addiction, such as the people you have hurt and the relationships you have lost. When you see these reminders, you may think you miss your old life, but in truth, it only brought you misery and hardship.

Accept the notion that you are constructing a new, healthier version of yourself with no room for the things of the past.

When you're feeling provoked, having a substitute habit, like going to a yoga class or taking a lengthy bath, can be beneficial. You might also be able to resist these temptations if you say happy mantras or do relaxation exercises. Work with your counselor or therapist to come up with extra strategies for dealing with these reminders.

E. Festive Occasions

Positive events, such as birthdays and holidays, can also serve as triggers. You may feel content, in control, and certain that you can handle one drink, one cigarette, or one light flirtation with the gorgeous stranger. But will you be able to keep it under control?

Addicts frequently lose their ability to recognize when it is time to stop. As a result, one drink could turn into a binge. Alternatively, buying one unnecessary new pair of shoes could lead to a shopping binge.

Having a friend can help if you are at risk of falling back into old habits. If you start to relapse, find someone you trust and respect to gently but forcefully encourage you to quit what you're doing.

Avoid entering into circumstances where you are at high risk of relapsing on your own. You may be amazed at how quickly your determination and good intentions fade once the party begins.

Make a strategy with your counselor or therapist to deal with the temptations that come with fun events like parties, weddings, and holidays. You are more prone to relapse if you enter the scenario unprepared.

How To Create A Relapse Prevention Plan

Managing anxiety or any other mental health disorder requires a plan to keep from falling back into old habits. It is a proactive approach that helps individuals identify and manage their triggers, warning signs, and potential challenges, to prevent relapse and maintain their recovery. Here are the steps to creating a relapse prevention plan:

A. **Identify triggers**: It's essential to be aware of the situations, thoughts, or events that can trigger anxiety symptoms. Some common triggers are stress, changes in routines, and traumatic events.

B. **Develop coping strategies**: Identify healthy coping mechanisms that work best for you, such as deep breathing exercises, meditation, exercise, and talking to someone.

C. **Create a support network**: Make sure to have a supportive network of family, friends, and professionals who you can turn to for help and support.

D. **Learn about your disorder**: Get informed about your anxiety disorder and how it can affect you. Understanding the condition can help you develop a better prevention plan.

E. **Plan for crises**: Identify the signs of an impending crisis and have a plan in place to handle it. For example, having a trusted friend or family member to talk to or a specific relaxation technique you can use.

F. **Practice self-care**: Regular self-care activities, such as exercise, healthy eating, and getting enough sleep, can help prevent relapse and maintain your recovery.

G. **Review and adjust**: Regularly evaluate your relapse prevention plan and adjust it as needed. Make sure to incorporate any new triggers or coping strategies that you discover.

Having a well-thought-out relapse prevention plan can give you the tools and confidence to manage your anxiety disorder and maintain your recovery over the long term.

Top Ten (10) Tips To Preventing Relapse From Drug Addiction

Everyone in recovery from drug addiction is in danger of relapsing, regardless of how long it has been since they last used a narcotic. The National Institute on Drug Abuse says that addiction is a disease that causes people to use drugs over and over again, usually despite bad effects. This causes long-term changes in the brain.

Addiction is a chronic and relapsing illness. This means that, like other disorders such as hypertension and asthma, there is no cure. Relapse is a typical feature of all chronic disorders, including addiction. According to studies, relapse rates for substance use disorders range between 40 and 60 percent.

If you are in recovery from a substance use disease and relapse, you have not failed. It does not invalidate your prior efforts to remain drug-free, nor does it imply that whatever treatment program you attended was ineffective. But that doesn't mean you should use it as an excuse to keep consuming drugs.

Although there is no cure for addiction, you can take steps to prevent relapse. You have to be proactive and keep at it if you want to stop the negative effects of addiction on your brain. There are numerous tools available to assist you in your long-term recovery path. These suggestions can help you stay clean and sober if you incorporate them into your treatment. (Though this applies to those challenged by drug addiction, these tips can be applied in all challenging situations.)

A. Begin With A Comprehensive Addiction Treatment Program

It is difficult to break the pattern of addiction on your own. If you've struggled to quit using on your own, you're not alone. When it comes to getting clean, addiction treatment is a terrific place to start. It puts you in a place where you can focus all of your energy on building a solid foundation for long-term recovery and avoiding relapse.

Depending on your requirements, there are numerous addiction treatment programs to choose from. There is a program for you, from detox to inpatient institutions to outpatient programs. Individual and group therapy, educational programs, and experiential treatment choices all work together to help you learn to live a drug-free life.

B. Complete Your Treatment Program Completely

Attending your treatment program the entire time may seem obvious to some, but it is a vital aspect of preventing relapse. People who leave therapy early, against medical advice, jeopardize their recovery. Even if you don't entirely love some aspects of addiction therapy, there is always something to learn and take away from them.

The amount of time and effort you put into treatment determines the pace of your recovery. You are not giving yourself the best chance to stay sober if you merely put in a modest amount of effort or exit your program early. Take advantage of any opportunity to attend treatment and make the most of the program that is available to you.

C. Create And Implement An Aftercare Strategy.

You'll sit down with your counselor or case manager near the end of your therapy to create an aftercare plan. When you finish your program and leave the treatment center, you will follow a plan for help called "aftercare." One of the best ways to prevent a recurrence is to stick to your treatment plan.

Most aftercare plans include some kind of outpatient program or drug and alcohol treatment. Some include attending 12-step meetings or residing in a sober living facility. The details of your aftercare plan will depend on your facility's requirements and services.

D. Create A Support Network With Whom You Can Stay In Touch Following Treatment.

Trying to stay clean and avoid relapse on your own is a challenging task. When you don't have a support network to hold you accountable, it's easier to relapse. When you're feeling isolated and pushed by the pressures of drug-free living, it's helpful to have a support network to whom you can turn.

Group therapy may be part of your recovery plan, which is a good place to start. Choose a few folks from your group with whom you'd like to spend time outside of therapy. When you're having a hard time outside of group hours, exchange phone numbers and reach out to one another.

E. Locate A Therapist To Provide Continued Individual Counseling

If your plan for aftercare doesn't include ongoing therapy, you may want to get help on your own. It is helpful to stay in touch with a counselor or therapist who knows how hard it is to live a life in recovery.

Therapy provides a secure space for you to work through current concerns as well as issues from your past that you did not get to work with in treatment. If you can keep going to therapy after treatment, you will be well on your way to not relapsing.

F. Attend 12-Step Meetings Or Other Forms Of Recovery Help

12-step meetings and other recovery support organizations put you in a room with individuals who understand your problems. There are support groups for each issue, from drugs and alcohol to gambling and overeating. Some people dislike the 12-step method of recovery; thus, groups such as SMART Recovery or Refuge Recovery may be beneficial in preventing recurrence.

G. Take Up A New Hobby Or Reconnect With An Old One

Only when you get clean do you realize how time-consuming it is to live a drug-addicted existence. The majority of your time is spent either under the influence of drugs or trying to come up with the money to acquire more drugs. When you remove substances from the equation, you have a lot of free time.

Idle time is not the best thing to do in the early stages of rehabilitation. If you want to avoid relapsing, spend your time finding new hobbies you enjoy or rediscovering ones that addiction has taken away from you. Cook a new recipe, attend a concert with sober friends, or join a slow-pitch softball league. There are numerous alternatives to using drugs to pass time.

H. Activate Your Muscle

Depression and anxiety are frequent problems in the early weeks and months after rehabilitation. It takes time to acclimate to your new life without the use of medications to mask your emotions. Exercise is a terrific way to enhance your energy and manage your mood by releasing endorphins in your brain. There's certain to be a way to get your body moving that you'll enjoy, whether it's walking, jogging, yoga, riding, swimming, lifting weights, or something else.

I. Maintain A Journal

Journaling is an excellent multipurpose tool for preventing relapse. Keep track of your moods, items that entice you to use, and enjoyable ways to spend your time in your notebook. Keeping a journal is a great way to look back on your recovery journey, think about your goals, and come up with a plan for how to reach your goals.

J. Do Not Be Afraid To Seek Assistance

Asking for help is not always easy, but if you want to avoid relapse, you must learn how to do it. This could include contacting your case manager or therapist, as well as your recovery support group or another group of friends. Perhaps you could try a self-help recovery program or a 12-step program.

It may be challenging at first, but it becomes simpler with practice. You are not alone in your struggle to live a drug-free life. The more you reach out to people and seek support along the path, the more likely you are to achieve long-term recovery.

How To Develop Healthy Coping Mechanisms To Deal With Triggers

In order to deal with triggers in a healthy way, you need to come up with ways to handle the strong feelings and thoughts that may come up. Some coping mechanisms include:

A. **Mindfulness and relaxation techniques**: Mindfulness, deep breathing, and progressive muscle relaxation can help reduce anxiety and calm the body when faced with a trigger.
B. **Exercise**: Regular physical activity can help reduce stress and anxiety, and improve overall well-being.
C. **Reframing thoughts**: Challenging negative thoughts and reframing them into positive ones can help reduce the impact of a trigger.
D. **Positive self-talk**: Encouraging oneself with positive affirmations and self-talk can help reduce the impact of a trigger.

E. **Connecting with others**: Talking to friends, family, or a therapist can help provide support and reduce feelings of isolation.

F. **Distraction techniques**: Engaging in activities that distract from the trigger, such as reading, watching a movie, or listening to music, can help reduce anxiety.

G. **Journaling**: Writing down thoughts and feelings can help process emotions and provide insight into triggers.

It is important to find what works best for each individual and to have a variety of coping mechanisms to choose from when faced with a trigger.

The Importance Of Self-Care In Avoiding Relapse

Self-care is a crucial component of avoiding relapse for those with anxiety disorders. Regular self-care activities, like exercise, mindfulness practices, and healthy eating, can help you stay physically and emotionally healthy, reduce stress, and stop symptoms from starting.

Also, doing things that make you happy and fulfilled, like hobbies or spending time with people you care about, can improve your overall mood and strength, making it easier to deal with any triggers that come up.

Setting aside time for self-care is important because not doing so can lead to burnout and make it harder to deal with symptoms. People with anxiety disorders can stay on the path to recovery and avoid relapse by making and sticking to a self-care routine.

How To Manage Stress And Maintain A Healthy Lifestyle To Prevent Relapse

Those with anxiety disorders must learn to deal with stress and live a healthy life in order to avoid relapse. Here are some tips to help:

A. **Exercise regularly**: Regular physical activity, such as going for a walk, jog, or engaging in any other form of physical activity, can help reduce stress and improve overall health.

B. **Practice good sleep habits**: Getting adequate, quality sleep is crucial in managing stress and preventing relapse. Aim for 7-9 hours of sleep per night and establish a regular sleep routine.

C. **Eat a balanced diet**: A balanced diet that is rich in fruits, vegetables, and whole grains can help improve physical and emotional well-being. Avoid processed and sugary foods, as these can exacerbate symptoms of anxiety.

D. **Reduce caffeine and alcohol consumption**: These substances can increase stress and trigger symptoms of anxiety.

E. **Practice relaxation techniques**: Techniques such as deep breathing, progressive muscle relaxation, and mindfulness can help calm the mind and reduce stress.

F. **Connect with others**: Having strong social support can help reduce stress and prevent relapse. Connecting with friends, family, and support groups can provide a sense of community and help build resilience.

G. **Engage in leisure activities**: Engaging in activities you enjoy, such as reading, gardening, or playing a sport, can help reduce stress and improve your overall mood.

It's important to remember that everyone's experience with anxiety is unique, and what works for one person may not work for another. It's important to find what works best for you and be patient with the process. By adding these ways to deal with stress to your daily routine, you can help stop relapses and stay free of anxiety for a long time.

How To Recognize And Avoid High-Risk Situations

Recognizing and staying away from high-risk situations is an important part of keeping anxiety disorders from coming back. High-risk situations are those that can increase the likelihood of a relapse, and it is important to be aware of these triggers in order to avoid them. Some common high-risk situations for anxiety disorders include:

- Stressful life events, such as job loss, financial problems, or relationship issues
- Substance abuse, including alcohol or drugs
- Lack of sleep or poor sleep quality
- Physical health issues, such as illness or injury
- Negative self-talk or negative thought patterns
- Isolation and loneliness
- Excessive exposure to technology or media

Self-care and living a healthy life are important if you want to avoid high-risk situations. This means getting regular exercise, eating a healthy diet, getting enough sleep, and spending less time with technology and other sources of stress. It might also help to find and deal with any underlying psychological or emotional problems that might be causing anxiety.

It is also important to have a strong support network, including friends, family, or a therapist, who can provide support and encouragement during difficult times. If you can't avoid a high-risk situation, having a plan for dealing with stress and anxiety can help you stay on track. This could mean doing things like practicing mindfulness or deep breathing, or reaching out to a trusted friend or therapist for help.

Recognizing and Managing Co-Occurring Disorders That May Contribute to Relapse

When a person has both a mental health disorder and a drug use disorder at the same time, they are said to have co-occurring disorders. When it comes to anxiety, co-occurring disorders can include depression, drug abuse, or other mental health problems. It is important to recognize these disorders and manage them effectively to prevent relapse.

Treatment for co-occurring disorders often involves a combination of therapy and medication. Cognitive-behavioral therapy (CBT) or dialectical behavior therapy (DBT) can be effective in addressing both the anxiety and the co-occurring disorder. Medications, such as antidepressants or mood stabilizers, may also be prescribed to manage the symptoms of co-occurring disorders.

People with co-occurring disorders can also manage their symptoms and avoid relapse by learning healthy ways to deal with stress and doing self-care activities like exercise and mindfulness. Building a strong support network, including by attending support groups and reaching out to loved ones, can also be beneficial in managing co-occurring disorders and maintaining long-term recovery.

How To Recognize And Manage The Signs Of Impending Relapse And Seek Help Quickly

Recognizing the signs of a possible relapse and getting help right away is an important part of a plan to stop relapses. Some common signs of an impending relapse may include:

- A return of anxiety or other symptoms of your condition
- Increased stress levels or changes in stressors
- Avoidance behaviors, such as withdrawing from activities or avoiding certain places or people
- Changes in sleep patterns, such as difficulty sleeping or increased fatigue
- Increased use of drugs or alcohol
- A decrease in self-care practices, such as exercise, healthy eating, and socializing.

If you notice any of these signs, it's important to reach out to a trusted friend, family member, or therapist for support. It's also important to stay engaged in your recovery program, such as by attending therapy or support groups, practicing relaxation and stress-management techniques, and maintaining a healthy lifestyle. If you need to, you may also want to think about changing the way you take your medications or getting more medical or mental health care. The key is to be proactive and take steps to prevent relapse as soon as possible.

CONCLUSION

In conclusion, overcoming anxiety disorders is a challenging but achievable goal. By understanding the causes and symptoms of anxiety and using effective coping strategies, individuals can successfully manage stress and worry.

Managing anxiety involves making a personal plan, setting goals that can be reached, building a support network, and taking care of yourself. Relapse prevention is also an important part of getting over an anxiety disorder. People can lower their risk of relapse by figuring out what sets them off, avoiding high-risk situations, and coming up with healthy ways to deal with stress.

With proper support and the right tools, individuals can successfully overcome anxiety disorders and lead a fulfilling, stress-free life. This practical guide gives a full look at the strategies and techniques that are needed to deal with anxiety disorder and helps people take charge of their mental health.